Cut It Out

Cut It Out

The C-Section Epidemic in America

Theresa Morris

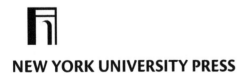

NEW YORK UNIVERSITY PRESS

New York and London

NEW YORK UNIVERSITY PRESS
New York and London
www.nyupress.org

References to Internet websites (URLs) were accurate at the time of writing. Neither the author nor New York University Press is responsible for URLs that may have expired or changed since the manuscript was prepared.

Library of Congress Cataloging-in-Publication Data
Morris, Theresa, 1956–
Cut it out : the C-section epidemic in America / Theresa Morris.
pages cm   Includes bibliographical references and index.
ISBN 978-0-8147-6411-4 (cl : alk. paper)
1. Cesarean section.   2. Cesarean section—Prevention.   3. Surgical
indications.   4. Women—Health and hygiene.   I. Title.
RG761.M67   2013
618.8'6—dc23   2013015226

New York University Press books are printed on acid-free paper, and their binding materials are chosen for strength and durability. We strive to use environmentally responsible suppliers and materials to the greatest extent possible in publishing our books.

Manufactured in the United States of America
10 9 8 7 6 5 4 3 2 1
Also available as an ebook

For Tim and our kiddos, Ben and Allie

Contents

Acknowledgments

I owe thanks and appreciation to many people who have helped me along the way with this project. I owe the most thanks to my husband, Tim, and our son, Ben, and daughter, Allie, for putting up with all of the time and attention I gave to the project. I have always felt a challenge in balancing competing demands—family, teaching, research, writing—and I know I have not always been successful at this balance. Thank you, Tim, Ben, and Allie, for being understanding and giving me time to think and write and think some more. If it weren't for you, Ben and Allie, I never would have become fascinated with the topic of birth. It was never a big interest of mine until your births.

I am deeply indebted to the maternity providers who took time to speak to me so honesty and candidly about the c-section rate. This was uncompensated time taken out of their busy schedules. Their willingness to be interviewed speaks to their commitment to women's health. I also thank all the women who allowed me a glimpse into their birth experiences.

I am fortunate to have worked with a number of smart, talented, and energetic undergraduate students. Molly Fitzgerald, Sophia Melograno, Jennifer Paluso, and Lee Ziesing conducted the interviews of postpartum women. Erin Flanagan, Elizabeth Gromisch, Sarah Quirk, Mary (Molly) Rose, Mia Schulman, Kimberly Shannon, and Valerie Small worked tirelessly on various aspects of this project. Financial support from Trinity College allowed me to hire many of these students.

Many people have supported this project by talking with me, asking and answering questions, and challenging me in critical ways to think about my research differently, including Karen Bayne, Danielle Bessett, LaDonna Boeckman, John Boies, Sherry Bruening, Pam Hunter-Holmes, Cathy Kamens, Susan Markens, Susan Masino, Jennifer Moller, Christine Morton, Harland Prechel, Louise Roth, Zena Ryder, Michael Sacks, Eileen Schopper, Carrie Lee Smith, and Tim Woods. John Boies, Sherry Bruening, Cathy Kamens, and Tim Woods read many drafts of the manuscript and provided priceless feedback. Their suggestions, no doubt, made the book much better. I owe a special thanks to John Boies, who helped create the figures in the book and who was a cheerleader of sorts for me throughout the entire writing and editing process. Cathy Kamens and Eileen Schopper tirelessly answered my many medical questions, and Libby Brinkley allowed me into the postpartum hospital unit she managed, in order for me to interview women.

I was also aided by a number of my colleagues at Trinity College. Alice Angelo endured endless interlibrary loan requests from me and filled them not only quickly but also patiently. Erin Valentino and Hebe Guardiola-Diaz taught me how better to manage my references. Rachael Barlow enthusiastically answered my questions about data and procured quantitative data whenever I asked. Cindy Butos was my go-to expert on tricky grammar questions.

I further wish to thank John Boies, Eduardo Bonilla-Silva, Adam Grossberg, Diane Pike, Harland Prechel, Michael Sacks, and David Wright for mentoring me at various stages of my academic career and my mother, Susan Morris; mother-in-law, Bobbie Woods; and good friend Liz Barry, who have been behind me all the way in writing this book.

Last but not least, I appreciate the confidence that my editor at NYU Press, Ilene Kalish, had in this project and in my ability to tell an important story.

Introduction

I hate c-sections. . . . There's more risk to the mother. It's more hassle for
me, takes more of my time, more postoperative recovery, more complications. I'd much rather deliver every baby vaginally if possible. There's one
reason why the c-section rate's up. The things that we [used to] do to help
make a vaginal delivery occur we're not allowed to do anymore.

        —Physician Jack Bianco

This book tells the story of how organizational changes constrain the decisions and behaviors of maternity providers and women in a way that
has resulted in an epidemic of cesarean sections—commonly, and in this
book, referred to as c-sections. Physician Bianco's statement about the c-
section rate aptly represents the ideas of many maternity care providers.[1]
They feel that they cannot do "the things" they used to do to facilitate a
vaginal birth. Such things include: monitoring the fetal heart rate during
labor intermittently rather than continuously; encouraging women with
twins and multiples, women who have had a previous c-section, or women
whose baby is presenting in a breech (head-up) position to have a vaginal
birth; and, most of all, optimistically waiting patiently for a vaginal birth
to happen. Not all maternity providers are as passionate as Doctor Bianco,
but his experience of having his decisions and actions constrained, of "not
being allowed" to make decisions or follow actions he thinks would lead to
a vaginal birth, are common, and maternity providers know this is making
the c-section rate climb. Yet they are making the best decisions they believe they can, given the pressures they face.

    Women giving birth in the United States face these constraints first-
hand. Indeed, my first experience giving birth is indicative of what many

women encounter today. I planned to give birth vaginally with no pain medications. I did all the things I thought would ensure that outcome. I attended childbirth education classes, ate a healthy diet, and regularly exercised, including doing tons of squats, which I read would help me push the baby out quickly. Everything was going as planned, and by my due date my cervix had dilated to four centimeters without any pain (a woman's cervix is considered fully dilated when it is ten centimeters in diameter). I was delighted when the physician overseeing my care told me that if anyone could give birth vaginally with no pain medication, it would be me, because my cervix had already dilated to four centimeters slowly and painlessly.

I went into labor exactly one day past my due date. At the hospital, a labor and delivery nurse performed an internal exam to access the dilation of my cervix. She found that my cervix was six centimeters dilated. Then she asked me an unexpected question: "Is this kid head down?" The physician overseeing my care was fortunately on call that day. She wheeled in a portable ultrasound machine, gelled up my belly, and ran the hand-held scanner over my swollen uterus to get a sense of the baby's position. The doctor sounded surprised when she told me the baby was in a frank-breech position (bottom down with legs straight up and feet laid against either side of his head). She then told me that I must have a c-section. I pleaded with her to help me have a vaginal birth, but she said a c-section was my only option—the baby was too big to turn to a head-down position (a procedure called external cephalic version or ECV) and she didn't deliver breech babies vaginally. I was shaken and upset by this turn of events. When I began to cry, the nurse scolded me: "Stop being a baby! Be thankful you are having a healthy baby!" I hastily signed a consent form for the surgery and was whisked to the operating room, where my son, eight pounds and seven ounces, was delivered by c-section. He had to stay in the hospital for six days because he had trouble breathing, a common problem for babies born by c-section because the amniotic fluid is not forced out of their lungs through the trip down their mother's birth canal, and his blood sugar was low.[2] We left the hospital a week later, somewhat battered and bruised by the ordeal. This was not a positive birth experience.

When I became pregnant with my daughter two years later, I was determined not to repeat that negative birth experience. I was committed to having a vaginal birth and to having more control over decisions that went into my care. I hired a birth doula (a professional labor assistant), researched having a vaginal birth after a c-section (VBAC), and wrote a birth plan.[3] Because my obstetrician was worried about the risk of uterine rupture (a small but known risk of laboring with a scarred uterus from a previous c-section) and, likely, perceived litigation risks, she was luke-warm about my plans and would have preferred that I schedule a repeat c-section, but I pressed on. The risk of a uterine rupture for a woman with one prior c-section is less than 1 percent, and maternal and fetal outcomes for women attempting VBAC are equivalent to the outcomes of women attempting a vaginal birth for the first time.[4] I felt secure in my decision.

After a short, five-hour, unmedicated labor in which I had to vigilantly refuse pain medications, IV fluids, and an internal fetal monitor, I gave birth to my daughter vaginally. Compared to my first birth, this was an incredibly empowering experience. But the enabling power of the birth was overshadowed by the struggle—in receiving support from maternity providers, staying free of interventions in the hospital, and having control over my labor and my daughter's birth.

Many of the women featured in these pages tell similar stories of feeling a lack of control during labor and birth. Cecelia was induced and had a vaginal delivery, but her doctor cut an episiotomy (where a woman's perineum is cut to enlarge the vaginal opening) without her consent. She told us, "They didn't inform [me] that [an episiotomy] was going on, which I thought they'd say, 'Can we cut you or do you just want to tear naturally?' I just sort of assumed someone would ask [me], and no one did." Another woman, Denise, had hoped to avoid having epidural anesthesia. When she became vocal during her labor, a common way women who are not medicated deal with labor pain, a nurse threatened her that if she did not get an epidural she was going to be taken to the operating room for a c-section. She explained, "The nurse asked me did I want to go have a c-section or get the epidural shot, and I ended up telling her that I wanted the epidural shot. So I ended up getting it." Vivian had a c-section because she was pregnant with twins, one who was presenting in a breech position. She was not given a choice to try a vaginal delivery because her physician preferred a c-section in this situation. She reports, "I was pregnant with twins. And it was a scheduled c-section, because [one of the twins] was not head down. And so when they're not both head down, they make you, my office feels more comfortable doing a c-section."

My birth experiences and the stories of women lacking control in birth piqued my interest in studying birth, in particular the increasing c-section rate. As I delved into my study, I developed a sense of empathy for maternity providers and began to see my experience through a different lens. The perspective I developed as a woman who gave birth in hospitals in the United States was that my choices were constrained. Yet what became clear to me in doing this research is that it is not only women who have their choices limited. Rather, the crux of this problem, and indeed I do see the increasing c-section rate as a problem, is that organizations determine the choices of women *and maternity providers*, and these constraints lead to an exceedingly high c-section rate, which in 2011 was an alarming 32.8 percent, a 50 percent increase in just the past decade.[5] In this book, I draw on intensive interviews I conducted with women, all of whom had given birth just a day before their interviews, and with maternity providers to examine an important question: if most women do not want or choose c-section and most maternity providers claim not to prefer c-section over vaginal birth, why has there been an astronomical increase in the c-section rate in the Untied States? This book will answer that question.[6]

Birth Patterns in the United States

It is important, first, to understand how birth happens in the United States and to become familiar with several terms used throughout the book.[7] Although this may come as a surprise, documenting birth trends in the United States is rather challenging due to how data on birth are collected. In 2003, Health and Human Services Secretary Tommy G. Thompson approved changes to the birth certificate form but did not require a uniform date for when states must adopt the revised birth certificate form. By 2010, thirty-three states had adopted the new certificate, while twenty-seven states were still using the 1989 version of the birth certificate form.[8] The problem this has created for researchers is that data collected on the revised birth certificate form are not always comparable to the data collected on the unrevised birth certificate form. This leaves researchers, including myself, in a quandary because some trends cannot be documented nationally since the two different birth certificate forms require different kinds of information and also because some data are not comparable year to year.[9]

I will walk readers through the existing knowledge of birth trends, sometimes drawing on national birth certificate data and other times drawing on the only comprehensive information of women's birth experiences in the United States that exists, the Listening to Mothers II survey in which a representative sample of women who gave birth in the United States in 2005 were asked about their labor and birth experiences. For the sake of brevity, I will refer to this survey as LTMII.[10] This survey also asked women many more questions about their labor and birth than are covered in the birth certificate form and is, thus, the most comprehensive information we have on women's actual birth experiences.

To begin, in 2011 32.8 percent of women who gave birth in the United States had a c-section.[11] We know from the LTMII survey that about half of all c-sections are performed on women who had a previous c-section.[12] In the sample of women to whom we spoke, 37 percent had a c-section, and 42 percent of these c-sections were performed on women who had a previous c-section. Repeat c-section is almost always scheduled ahead of time, and almost all scheduled c-sections are repeat c-sections.[13] A small percentage of women who have a scheduled c-section have not had a previous a c-section. In the LTMII survey, 90 percent of these women scheduled the c-section because a maternity provider recommended it for a medical reason.[14] The most common reasons were: the positioning of the baby, such as breech (head up), transverse (sideways), or posterior (face up) (25 percent); the maternity provider's belief that the baby was too big for a vaginal birth (12 percent); a problem with the placenta, such as the placenta covering the cervix (placenta previa) or having attached too deeply into the uterine wall (placenta accreta) (3 percent); or the mother's having a medical condition that precluded a vaginal birth (less than 1 percent).[15]

I describe in the following paragraphs what a typical c-section is like, although I should be clear that there are variations on a c-section procedure and, thus, some women will find that they had a different experience than exactly what I describe.

C-sections take place in an operating room.[16] If the woman has not already received an epidural during labor, she is typically given regional anesthesia, either an epidural or spinal. In an emergency a woman may be placed under general anesthesia. After the anesthesiologist administers the anesthesia, a nurse scrubs the woman's abdomen, places a catheter in her bladder, and drapes her abdomen to create a sterile field. The nurse tapes the woman's arms down by her sides, or sometimes straight out in a T formation, starts an IV, and attaches instruments to the woman's skin to monitor her vital signs. If the woman has regional anesthesia, a support person is usually allowed in the room. He or she sits next to the woman's head, and the anesthesiologist sits on the other side.

Surgery begins with the obstetrician making an incision in the woman's skin, typically just above the pubic bone. This type of incision is sometimes referred to as a bikini cut because the cut is so low that a woman should be able to wear a bikini without the scar being visible. The incision is almost always horizontal. The obstetrician may make a vertical incision in an emergency, but it is rare for a vertical incision to be performed in nonemergency situations. The obstetrician then locates the uterus and makes a uterine incision, usually horizontal. The direction of cut on the uterus is important because uterine rupture in subsequent pregnancies is much less likely to happen if the uterus is cut horizontally rather than vertically. The incision in the skin and the incision in the uterus may not be the same; that is, one may be vertical and the other horizontal. The obstetrician reaches into the uterus, maneuvers the baby out, and then clamps and cuts the umbilical cord. A nurse takes the baby, suctions her mouth and nose, assesses her breathing, and wraps her in a warmed towel. Next, the obstetrician manually removes the placenta and any remaining blood clots and placental tissue from the uterus and stitches the uterine incision closed. The obstetrician finishes by closing the skin incision with either stitches or staples. An uncomplicated c-section typically takes around an hour. Recovery from a c-section is not unlike recovery from any major abdominal surgery. It takes about six weeks for women to feel well enough to resume normal, everyday activities.

Labor and vaginal birth are much more varied than are c-sections. The labor and birth of women who attempt a vaginal birth (84 percent of women in the LTMII survey) encompass three stages.[17] The first stage is what we typically think of as "labor" and is the process of the cervix dilating to ten centimeters in diameter. The second stage is when the baby is born. Finally, the third stage is the expulsion of the placenta from the uterus—the placenta detaches from the uterine wall, and the woman pushes it out through her vagina. In the following paragraphs I discuss all three stages and use national data to describe trends in labor and birth. Because 98.8 percent of American births happen in hospitals, I focus on hospital births.[18]

According to the LTMII survey, 58 percent of women who attempt a vaginal birth arrive at a hospital in labor.[19] A nurse performs a cervical exam to see how dilated, or open, and how effaced, or thinned out, the woman's cervix is and to check the position of the baby. A nurse also monitors the baby's heart rate with a handheld Doppler or with an electronic fetal monitor to evaluate whether the baby is under stress.[20] A physician or midwife then makes the decision about whether to admit the woman and transfer her to a labor and delivery room or whether to send her home with instructions to come back when the labor is further progressed. Sometimes women want to be admitted even if they are in very early labor—hospitals and maternity providers vary on whether they allow this—and sometimes maternity providers admit all women who come to the hospital regardless of whether they are in active labor.

Once a decision has been made to admit the woman as a patient to the hospital, she is asked to sign an informed consent form for labor and birth, which covers interventions that might happen in birth, excluding c-section and anesthesia, which have separate consent forms. A nurse will ask her to change into a hospital gown and place an IV or, less likely, a hep- or saline-lock, a small tube connected to a vein in the arm that enables an IV to be started quickly but still allows the woman to move freely about the room while in labor. Overall, 83 percent of women in the LTMII survey had an IV during labor.[21]

Forty-one percent of women in the LTMII survey who attempted a vaginal birth had their labors artificially started, a process referred to as the induction of labor.[22] In my sample, a nearly identical 41.3 percent of women were induced. Induction is typically a scheduled procedure. A woman who has a scheduled induction arrives at the hospital at an agreed-on time, signs a consent form, changes into a hospital gown, and is connected to an IV. If her cervix is not effaced or thinned out, indicating it is favorable for induction, a physician or midwife gives her a drug to "ripen" her cervix, such as Dinoprostone (Cervidil, Prepidil, or Prostin E2) or Misoprostol (Cytotec), which a physician or midwife inserts near her cervix. Once her cervix is effaced, or if her cervix was effaced when she arrived for induction, the woman is typically given oxytocin (Pitocin), a drug administered through the IV that stimulates uterine contractions. Pitocin may also be given at any point in labor to augment a woman's labor if the contractions are deemed inadequate. Fifty-five percent of women in the LTMII survey received Pitocin augmentation at some point during their labors.[23] In my sample of women, 52.4 percent of women said they had received Pitocin augmentation at some point during their labors.

Sometimes induction fails to start a woman's labor. In such a case the woman may be sent home and asked to come back when labor begins or to try the induction process again later, or she may be told that she needs a c-section. For example, twenty-five-year-old Roxanne had a c-section after her induction with Cytotec and Pitocin failed. Nearly twenty-four hours after the start of the induction process, she was only three to four centimeters dilated. Here's how she described her reaction to this news: "I was like, 'Are you fricking kidding me?' . . . She [my obstetrician] said . . . 'At this point we can't give you any more Pitocin. We're at the max. You know, we've done everything we could.' So I ended up with a c-section."

In either an induced labor or a labor that starts spontaneously, nurses monitor the baby's heart rate and the woman's uterine contraction patterns. Maternity providers want most to know how the baby's brain is faring in the labor process. However, because the health of the baby's brain cannot easily be assessed during labor, the baby's heart rate has become the focus. The goal of monitoring the baby's heart rate is to prevent lack of oxygen to the baby, called hypoxia, which can lead to physical or mental disabilities and, at the most extreme, death.[24] The baby's heart rate is assessed with one of two different technologies.[25] Nurses may use a handheld Doppler. This type of monitoring is referred to as auscultation and is performed intermittently, typically every thirty minutes during active labor and every five minutes when the woman is pushing.[26] When a nurse uses a Doppler device to monitor the baby's heart rate, she palpates, or feels, the woman's abdomen to determine the strength and timing of contractions.

It is much more likely for nurses to monitor the baby's heart rate and uterine contraction pattern electronically with cardiotocography (CTG), commonly referred to as electronic fetal monitoring (EFM). Current survey data of women who give birth in the United States suggest that 93 percent of women have continuous electronic fetal monitoring in their labors, making it the most common obstetric procedure performed in the country.[27] CTG measures uterine contractions electronically with a pressure button attached with a band that is placed around a woman's abdomen.[28] The baby's heart rate is measured with another band placed around the woman's abdomen (external monitoring) or by placing an electrode into the baby's scalp (internal monitoring). External CTG can be used to check the baby's heart rate continuously or intermittently, while internal monitoring is used only continuously.

CTG units record the baby's heart rate and uterine contraction tracings on a paper called a strip. Uterine contractions are monitored for their strength, duration, and length between contractions, while the baby's heart rate is monitored for frequency and variation, with particular attention paid to decelerations or slowdowns, often referred to as decels.[29] A baby's heart rate frequency is considered normal when it is between 110 and 160 beats per minute. Bradychardia is defined as a baseline heart rate less than 110 beats per minute, and tachycardia is defined as a baseline heart rate over 160 beats per minute.[30] The baseline heart rate is established over a ten-minute period where there is consistency in the heart rate for at least two minutes.[31]

Two heart-rate frequency patterns concern maternity providers. The first pattern is referred to as late decelerations. Late decelerations happen when the baby's heart rate falls at the beginning of a contraction and returns to its baseline after the contraction has ended.[32] Late decelerations concern providers because they might indicate that the baby or the placenta is compromised. Blood vessels lay within an intricate weave of uterine muscles, and when the uterus contracts, much of the blood flow to the placenta is cut off, decreasing the oxygen supply to the baby. If the baby and placenta are healthy, the baby can sustain this loss of oxygen with stores of energy. However, if the baby is not responding well to labor or is not healthy or if the placenta is not strong enough, the baby cannot maintain her oxygen level when the placental blood supply is reduced, resulting in heart-rate declarations with contractions. Late decelerations are considered recurrent if they occur with at least 50 percent of contractions over a twenty-minute window.[33]

The other type of heart-rate deceleration that is concerning to maternity providers is referred to as variable decelerations. Variable decelerations are not related to the timing of uterine contractions—they happen almost randomly—and are typically due to the compression of the umbilical cord. Umbilical cord compression can be, but is not necessarily, caused by a prolapsed umbilical cord, a very serious condition in which the umbilical cord drops through the cervix. Umbilical cord prolapse is considered an obstetrical emergency necessitating an immediate c-section because the baby's head pushing against the cervix can cut off the baby's blood and oxygen supply. If the baby's heart rate has variable decelerations and cord prolapse is ruled out, the woman is usually asked to shift her position in an attempt to free the umbilical cord. Amnioinfusion may also be used to aid in this situation. In amnioinfusion a saline solution is added to the amniotic fluid by inserting a catheter (or tube) directly into the cervix. It is believed that adding fluid to the uterus may reduce pressure on the umbilical cord. Although research suggests this may be an effective way to alleviate umbilical cord compression, more research needs to be done to confirm this finding.[34] One study found that one-third of women who experience variable decelerations in their labors receive amnioinfusion.[35]

Nurses also monitor variability, or fluctuation, of the baby's heart rate with CTG. Variability is defined as absent, minimal (fewer than five beats per minute), moderate (between six and twenty-five beats per minute), or marked (more than 25 beats per minute).[36] Maternity providers are assured when babies have moderate variability in the heart rate. Minimal or marked heart rate variability could be, but is not necessarily, a sign of distress, while a persistent absence of variability is considered a reason for immediate delivery.

Maternity providers carefully monitor CTG tracings for problematic heart rate patterns because they worry that a problematic pattern may indicate injury to the baby, particularly cerebral palsy (a disability involving the central nervous system characterized by lack of control of body movement) or impending death.[37] CTG was commercially introduced in 1968 and was seen as a triumph because physicians thought it would more accurately monitor a baby's heart rate and prevent a baby's demise or disability. However, as logical as this sounds and as avid as their belief was, there is no empirical evidence that its use improves a baby's outcomes compared to intermittent auscultation using a handheld Doppler unit.[38] In fact, CTG has a 99.8 percent false positive rate, which means that the baby is fine 99.8 percent of the time in which the CTG strip looks problematic.[39] This almost unbelievable false positive rate is related to a little known fact: most cases of cerebral palsy are *not* linked to anything that happens during birth. For many years it was believed that cerebral palsy was caused by a lack of oxygen during birth. However, scientific evidence now suggests that, although lack of oxygen at birth is a possible cause of cerebral palsy, *most* cases of cerebral palsy are *not* linked to problems that occur during labor.[40]

Still, maternity providers have an overwhelming concern that lack of oxygen at birth may result in this disease and that they will be blamed for the negative birth outcome. Because of this concern, maternity providers watch carefully for "non-reassuring" heart beat patterns. If such a pattern is detected, maternity providers, primarily nurses and midwives, may perform amnioinfusion or may ask the woman to change positions or breathe oxygen to resolve it. If the woman is being induced or augmented with Pitocin, the drug might be turned down or off. If the baby's non-reassuring heart beat pattern does not resolve, the woman will be rushed to the operating room for a c-section. The reason for the c-section will be listed as "fetal distress." Twenty-five percent of primary (or first) c-sections are done for this reason.[41] In the sample of women I studied, 27 percent of women with unplanned c-sections gave this as the reason for their c-section. A typical way women talked about this is demonstrated in Melissa's description about why she had a c-section: "They determined that the baby's heart rate was just too variable and got too many dips, and I ended up having to do an emergency cesarean." This all helps to explain why the use of continuous CTG increases a woman's chance of having a c-section.[42]

Another disadvantage of monitoring a woman's labor with continuous CTG is that it typically confines her to bed because the electrical cord of the unit reaches just a few feet. This restricts the woman's movement and her access to a shower or bath. Such restrictions can result in extraordinary discomfort for a laboring woman, who may need to shift positions or walk around to endure painful contractions over several hours. Movement and sitting in water are both natural ways women may use to deal with labor pains. Telemetry CTG units, which use radio waves or computer networks to remotely monitor contractions and the baby's heart rate, allow women freedom of movement, and some CTG telemetry units function in water. However, these units are not universally available to women, and nurses complain that they are difficult to use and must be constantly readjusted to assure accurate readings.

Partly, then, as a result of the nearly universal use of continuous CTG, most women (86 percent in the LTMII survey) receive pain medication during labor.[43] Epidural analgesia is the most common method of analgesic pain relief (analgesics relieve pain without the loss of consciousness)—71 percent of women in the LTMII survey who delivered vaginally had an epidural.[44] In the sample of women I studied, the use of epidurals was more common: 86 percent of women who attempted a vaginal birth had an epidural. About one in five women in the LTMII survey received narcotics through an IV, such as Demerol or Stadol, and 16 percent of women had both a narcotic and an epidural during labor.[45] It is common for women who have an epidural to be augmented with Pitocin because epidurals often slow down labor.[46] The prolonging effect of epidurals on labor is likely due to the "labor-slowing effects" of intravenous fluids.[47]

It may also occur that women who are augmented with Pitocin may be more likely to receive epidurals. Women often experience Pitocin contractions as more painful because contractions reach their peaks more quickly than natural contractions do.[48] Wanda, a first-time mother, described the pain she felt from Pitocin: "I'm twenty-two years old and [have] never [been] through this kind of pain before. . . . This is the worst, and I thought that when I went through the labor . . . that I was like wounded or something. . . . It was really painful."

Another common labor intervention, performed supposedly to speed labor, is to artificially rupture a woman's amniotic sac (or "membranes" or "bag of waters"). This procedure is called amniotomy or AROM (artificial rupture of membranes). Sixty-five percent of women in the LTMII survey had this intervention.[49] A smaller percentage of women in my sample,

49.2 percent, mentioned having their membranes ruptured. There is no evidence that amniotomy shortens the first stage of labor, and amniotomy is possibly linked to an increased risk of having a c-section.[50] In general, maternity providers like women to deliver within twenty-four hours of her amniotic sac rupturing (naturally or artificially) to prevent infection in the women or baby, which means that once amniotomy is performed, the clock starts ticking.

Women in labor typically do not eat (only 15 percent of women eat) or drink (only 43 percent of women drink) during labor in the hospital.[51] Sometimes a woman's not eating is due to her decreased appetite during labor, but more often it is due to maternity providers' and hospital administrators' concern with the risk of a woman's aspirating if she has an emergency c-section under general anesthesia. Aspiration is a known risk of general anesthesia because general anesthesia suppresses the normal gag reflex, which means that vomited food or gastric fluid from a woman's stomach may enter her lungs.[52] Not allowing women to drink during labor is almost certainly due to hospital restrictions, as women in labor often have insatiable thirst. This thirst is why women laboring in hospitals are so commonly seen sucking on ice chips—many hospital rules allow women to satisfy their thirst only with ice chips. Restricting women's access to food and drink during labor does not improve birth outcomes.[53] In fact, it is quite counterintuitive to deny women sustenance while they are engaged in an energy-draining process—labor and birth.

If a woman takes "too long" to dilate, typically defined as not dilating at the pace of one centimeter per hour, maternity providers may decide on a c-section. Maternity providers may not know why labor is stalled, or they may believe that it is due to a baby that is too big to descend into the birth canal. In such situations the reason for the surgery will be listed as "failure to progress" or "cephalic pelvic disproportion" (CPD). We know from the LTMII survey that 26 percent of primary c-sections are done because the labor takes too long, because the mother is exhausted, or because the maternity provider believes that the baby is too big.[54] In the sample of women I studied, this was a very common reason for a primary c-section—53 percent of women who had a primary c-section had it for failure to progress or for CPD. Christina had such an experience. After her cervix dilated to nine centimeters, she was told that her pelvis was too small to allow the baby to descend and dilate her cervix to ten centimeters: "They said the shape of the bone, I guess, sometimes is bigger, and sometimes they're smaller. I guess mine was smaller so I couldn't have him through there." Likewise, twenty-seven-year-old Jessica says, "I got to eight centimeters and they checked and . . . it just wasn't going to happen. . . . Then my doctor just said, 'You know what? This [c-section] is the way we have to go.'"

Once a maternity provider determines that a woman's cervix is ten centimeters in diameter (usually by an internal exam—81 percent of women in the LTMII survey had at least one internal exam), women begin the second stage of labor—pushing the baby out.[55] Most women in the LTMII survey pushed on their backs or propped up in a semi-sitting position (92 percent).[56] Some women were aided in a variety of ways. The physician or midwife enlarged the vaginal opening by cutting through the woman's perineum, a procedure called an episiotomy (25 percent), the physician, midwife, or nurse pushed on the woman's belly to help the baby move down (17 percent), or the physician used a vacuum or forceps (7 percent) to help pull the baby out.[57]

Most maternity providers become concerned if a woman pushes for longer than two or three hours. One of the main concerns maternity providers have with slow delivery is the small risk of shoulder dystocia, which occurs when a baby's head is delivered vaginally but her shoulders get stuck behind the woman's pubic bone. There is no valid way of predicting shoulder dystocia—this is a random event—and it occurs in only 2 percent of all births.[58] But when shoulder dystocia does occur it is an emergency because the condition can result in injuries to the baby, the most common of which are clavicle (collarbone) fracture and brachial plexus injuries. (The brachial plexus nerves go from the spine to the shoulder, arm, and hand and control the hand, wrist, elbow, and shoulder.) Although extremely rare, shoulder dystocia can lead to fetal asphyxiation and death.[59] The occurrence of birth injury or death due to shoulder dystocia is slight. For example, brachial plexus injury occurs in less than one-third of one percent of all live births.[60] Research suggests, further, that more than four hundred c-sections would need to be performed to prevent one case of a lifelong brachial plexus injury.[61] But, if a woman is unable to push the baby out within a "reasonable" time, providers may worry that the baby is lodged and that a shoulder dystocia is inevitable. For example, Emily, a twenty-nine-year-old first-time mother, who pushed for only ten minutes before being told she needed a c-section, said, "I started pushing and basically I'm too small to deliver the baby, so they had to do an emergency c-section." The average length of the labor, including dilation and pushing time, is ten hours.[62]

The third stage of labor is when the placenta is expelled from the uterus. The uterus continues to contract until the placenta detaches from the uterine wall and the woman pushes it out. Breastfeeding the baby can hasten the delivery of the placenta because breastfeeding stimulates the body's release of oxytocin, which helps the uterus to contract and expel the placenta.[63] Nurses typically give women Pitocin (artificial oxytocin) either through an IV or as an injection to stimulate uterine contractions, although I do not have information on the percentage of women who receive Pitocin for this purpose.

According to the LTMII survey, 16 percent of women who attempt a vaginal birth have an unplanned c-section.[64] A c-section may be suggested at any point during the labor—if the CTG tracing is non-reassuring, if the woman's cervix dilates too slowly, if the baby seems too big, if the woman seems too small, if the woman pushes too long, and the list goes on. This book is about those 16 percent of women who have an unplanned c-section and the 16 percent of women who have a scheduled c-section—or the over 32 percent of pregnant women who have c-sections each year.

The Importance of This Research

As I began to explore c-sections as a sociological research topic, I found it to be one of ever more importance. Perhaps most notably, this trend stands in stark contrast to promoting the health of women and babies.[65] C-sections are associated with a higher risk of injury and death to women and babies than is vaginal birth.[66] The risks of c-sections have become better understood in the last decade, as researchers have been better able to compare vaginal births to c-sections. In the past, researchers were unable to separate out the outcomes of planned c-sections from unplanned c-sections. Thus, when women and babies fared more poorly in c-section births than in vaginal births, critics would argue that this difference was due to unplanned c-sections being performed in emergencies. Recent research, however, has separated out these births to better examine the outcomes of a planned c-section compared to the outcomes of a vaginal birth. Since 2006 several studies have been published that make clear that the outcomes of vaginal birth for women and babies are better than the outcomes of c-section, planned or unplanned.

In 2006, Catherine Deneux-Tharaux and colleagues published a study comparing maternal mortality (death) in France in vaginal deliveries, in c-sections that were performed after labor began (intrapartum), and in c-sections that were performed before labor began (prepartum).[67] By separating intrapartum c-sections and prepartum c-sections, the researchers hoped to get at the question of the safety of *planned* c-sections (i.e. prepartum c-sections). Deneux-Tharaux and colleagues removed from the analysis any women with risk factors that might predispose them to having a c-section or complications from a c-section. They found that maternal mortality was higher in c-sections than in vaginal deliveries by 3.3 to 3.6 times, and the difference between intrapartum and prepartum c-sections was not significant. In summary, the study found that women are more likely to die in a c-section than in vaginal birth, regardless of whether the surgery is planned.

In 2007 José Villar and colleagues published a well-designed study of births in Latin America and found that, taking out the effect of hospital setting and any risk factors the woman might have, planned c-sections were associated with higher rates of maternal morbidity (injury), mortality (death), and fetal mortality (death) than were planned vaginal births.[68] This World Health Organization (WHO)–supported study indicates that planned vaginal birth is safer than planned c-sections for women *and babies.*

Marian MacDorman and colleagues in a 2008 article compared neonatal mortality (death) rates in planned vaginal births and planned c-sections in the United States.[69] These researchers used an intention-to-treat research design, which deals with the problem of distinguishing outcomes of *planned* c-sections from outcomes of *unplanned* c-sections by separating births according to whether they were planned vaginal births or planned c-sections. If a woman plans a vaginal birth but has a c-section, her baby's data are still grouped with the planned vaginal birth group. The only births included in the planned c-section group are for women who planned to have a c-section. MacDorman and colleagues found a higher neonatal death rate in planned c-section births than in planned vaginal births, by a rate of 1.69–2.4 times, a clear indication that even if a c-section is planned, it is still less safe for the baby than is vaginal birth.

Other examples of how a c-section is riskier to women than a vaginal birth include research that shows that women who have a c-section face an increased risk of hysterectomy, rehospitalization, and prolonged pain.[70] Further, women who have a c-section are more likely than women who give birth vaginally to encounter infertility and troubles in future pregnancies, such as stillbirth, problems with the placenta, and uterine rupture.[71] These increased risks have not gone unnoticed by health insurance companies, some of which deny insurance coverage or charge higher premiums to women who have had a c-section unless the women are sterilized or are past their childbearing years.[72]

Further, a study by William M. Callaghan, Andreea S. Creanga, and Elena V. Kuklina published in November 2012 in *Obstetrics and Gynecology* examines severe maternal morbidity during delivery and postpartum hospitalizations in the United States. Although not specifically about morbidity risks of c-sections, the study finds that thirteen indicators of severe morbidity (e.g., shock, thrombotic embolism, and blood transfusion) more than doubled between 1998 and 2009, and women with at least one complication increased by two-thirds in the same period.[73] The authors write, "On an annual basis, with approximately 4,000,000 births in the United States, 129 episodes of severe maternal morbidity will affect approximately 52,000 women."[74] Clearly, more attention needs to be paid to this trend, which is surely at least partly due to the c-section epidemic.

Vaginal birth, then, is unquestionably safer for women and babies than are c-sections. The one issue that sometimes comes up in this discussion is a common belief that a vaginal birth is more likely than a c-section to damage a woman's pelvic floor muscles, leading to incontinence (an inability to control the discharge of urine or feces). Although more thorough research needs to be conducted on this question, current evidence does not support the claim that c-sections protect a woman's pelvic floor compared to vaginal birth.[75]

Beyond the risks posed to babies by c-section highlighted above, babies born by c-section also have increased risk of respiratory problems and future asthma and are at risk of being cut during the surgery.[76] Note, too, that although the c-section rate has increased steadily in the United States, the rates of cerebral palsy and shoulder dystocia have stayed the same.[77] In fact, research shows that hospitals with high c-section rates do not have better neonatal outcomes than do hospitals with low c-section rates, and this is the case for all types of hospitals.[78] In other words the health of newborns has not been improved by the epidemic of c-sections.

When c-sections are planned, there is a particular risk of a baby's being born prematurely because there is no way to know with absolute precision a baby's gestational age, measured as weeks since the start of the woman's last menstrual period. Babies delivered before forty weeks gestation have an increased risk of mortality (death) and morbidity (injury), and the rate of late-term prematurity, defined as babies born between thirty-four and thirty-seven weeks gestation, has been increasing since 2005.[79] This trend is at least partially tied to scheduled c-sections, largely because of dating errors (that is, believing, for example, a baby is thirty-eight weeks gestation when it is really thirty-seven weeks gestation).[80]

A second important reason to study the c-section epidemic is that the 2011 U.S. c-section rate of 32.8 percent, the most recent rate available, is more than double the maximum recommended rate of 15 percent proposed by the World Health Organization.[81] As shown in figure I.1, the c-section rate has soared from just over 5 percent in 1970 to almost 33 percent in 2011, and the rate has increased among women of all ages, races, and medical conditions and among babies of all gestational age.[82]

It is not a small matter for a country to so exceed this defined optimal c-section rate. According to the World Health Organization, countries with a c-section rate higher than 15 percent put women's lives at risk.[83] All of this may help to explain why the U.S. maternal mortality rate has increased an astounding 75 percent in the past twenty years from 12 per 100,000 live births in 1990 to 21 per 100,000 live births in 2010.[84] This rate is now higher than the maternal mortality rate of all of western Europe and also higher than the maternal mortality rate in countries such as Bosnia and Herzegovina (8 per 100,000 live births), Lithuania (8 per 100,000 live births), Serbia (12 per 100,00 live births), Croatia (17 per 100,000 live births), and Turkey (20 per 100,000 live births).[85]

Finally, unnecessary c-sections are a drain on the American economic system. Annual health care expenditures in the United States increased by over 1,000 percent between 1960 and 2006 (adjusted for inflation) to a whopping $2.1 trillion; c-sections contributed to this increase.[86] Childbirth is a significant part of health care expenditures in the United States. The most costly hospital condition for Medicaid and private insurers is "mother's pregnancy and delivery."[87] C-sections cost almost twice that of vaginal deliveries, and in 2008 there were 1.4 million c-sections performed at a cost of about $8.7 billion.[88] In a report on the costs of having a baby in the United States in 2010, researchers report that health care costs could be reduced by $5 billion if the c-section rate were reduced from 33 percent to 15 percent.[89]

Certainly some c-sections are necessary; c-sections can be a life-saving operation. For example, a woman whose placenta covers her cervix (placenta previa) must have a c-section. A woman who has a medical condition, such as a cardiac problem, that makes pushing a baby out risky, must have a c-section. Some babies do not tolerate labor and are compromised during the labor process, and some labors become obstructed. A c-section can be a life-saving operation in these situations. In fact, scholars estimate that countries with a c-section rate lower than 5 percent put women's health at risk.[90] This is the case in many underdeveloped countries, where

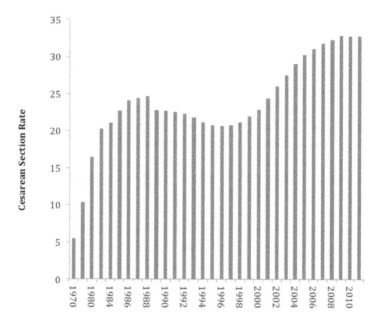

Figure I.1. U.S. Cesarean Section Rates, 1970–2011.

women die in childbirth every day because they do not have access to safe and timely c-sections.[91] In fact, one of the United Nations Millennium Development Goals is to reduce maternal mortality, and one way the United Nations proposes to do this is to increase women's access to skilled attendants at birth, which includes making sure that women have access to c-sections.[92] What this book explores is not why there are c-sections, but rather why there are *so many* c-sections in the United States.

Common Explanations for the C-Section Epidemic

It is commonly believed that physicians and pregnant women are responsible for the c-section epidemic. Explanations that focus on women or physician characteristics as related to c-sections inevitably put the blame of the increasing rate on one of these groups—physicians *cause* the increasing c-section rate, or women *cause* the increasing c-section rate. This finger pointing is common in the medical literature. For example, many explanations of the U.S. c-section rate focus on how individual characteristics of women affect their likelihood of having a c-section. This literature suggests that older women, larger women, women who gain excess weight in pregnancy, women of color, and women with private insurance are more likely to have a c-section.[93] However, focusing on the individual characteristics of women does not get us far in explaining the soaring c-section rate. The rate has gone up among all groups of women, and women have not changed so much in thirty years to suggest that one-third of women are now incapable of vaginal birth.

The hottest topic in terms of a woman's individual characteristics making her more likely to have a c-section is the focus on maternal request for c-sections, otherwise known as the "too posh to push" explanation in which wealthy, educated women "choose" medically unnecessary c-sections. It is important to debunk this myth because, although the too-posh-to-push explanation is commonly cited as a reason for the escalation of the c-section rate, there is no evidence to suggest it exists. The LTMII survey found that only 1 of the more than 1,300 (.08 percent) women surveyed who might have chosen a primary c-section instigated a request for a c-section with no medical indication.[94] Other studies have also questioned maternal request for c-sections being a significant trend.[95]

Research documenting an increase in maternal requests has also been questioned methodologically, particularly because it is very difficult to untangle whether women who have a c-section with no medical indication request the surgery or whether maternity providers recommend the surgery, as this information is not included on birth certificates.[96] In 2006 the U.S. National Institutes of Health held a State-of-the-Science meeting on maternal request for c-sections. Participants in the meeting witnessed incredible conflict, with some vociferously arguing that there was not sufficient evidence on the occurrence of maternal request for c-sections to justify a State-of-the-Science conference.[97] In short, there is little empirical evidence to support the "trend" of maternal request for c-sections.

Still, it is a common perception among U.S. obstetricians that maternal request is a driving force behind the increasing c-section rate. One study found that obstetricians commonly perceive that maternal request is a primary force behind the increasing c-section rate, even if they themselves have had no or few requests to perform a primary c-section with no medical indication.[98] Some scholars have suggested that pointing to maternal requests as one of the main contributors to the increasing c-section rate shifts the responsibility to women when, in fact, physicians are making the critical decision to perform a c-section.[99]

Further, NIH and ACOG have not taken a strong stand on the safety of c-sections without medical indication. In fact, although the evidence now points to vaginal birth as safer for women and babies than c-sections, planned or unplanned, ACOG's Committee on Ethics in 2008 stated that because the evidence of the safety of planned c-section versus planned vaginal birth is unclear, providers should evaluate risk of elective c-sections on a case-by-case basis.[100] This recommendation flies in the face of the research evidence. Because NIH and ACOG have given providers little direction on how to decide whether it is safer for a woman to give birth by a planned c-section or a planned vaginal delivery, maternity providers have been left to assess risk on their own, which, of course, is not an ideal situation. It allows for their own or collective biases, fears, and preferences to affect how risk is assessed and to transfer this perception to women.[101]

This leads me to the literature that focuses on the characteristics of the physicians in explaining the c-section rate. This literature suggests that physicians who graduate from medical programs outside the United States and physicians who use time management techniques during labor (being strict about the time a woman spends in any one stage of labor) have higher c-section rates, while physicians who use active labor management techniques (actively managing a woman's admission to the labor unit and progression in labor and intervening quickly when labor slows), allow women a trial of labor after a previous c-section, or who are family physicians, female physicians, or physicians with academic appointments have lower c-section rates.[102] This literature focuses, in general, on how training and location affects physicians' tolerance of labor and vaginal birth.

A Sociological Explanation of Cesarean Sections: The Meaning of Birth in Hospitals

A less-emphasized focus of the literature that examines c-sections looks at the effect of organizations such as hospitals and malpractice insurers on the c-section rate. This literature has found that teaching hospitals and health maintenance organizations (HMOs) have lower c-section rates, as do states with many HMOs.[103] In addition, studies have found a relationship between malpractice insurance premium increases and malpractice lawsuit experience and the increasing c-section rate.[104] The organizational scholars Elizabeth Goodrick and Gerald R. Salancik use c-sections as a case study to understand how uncertainty in the organizational environment may lead to hospitals having more discretion in decisions, such as the decision to perform a c-section.[105]

Although these studies allude to the importance of organizations, they are based on what Max Weber, a founder of sociology, refers to as a "direct understanding" of meaning.[106] In direct understanding, organizations are understood by observing organizational behavior—that is, how organizations act—but there is no attempt to understand how organizational behavior is linked to human behavior. In other words, the focus is not on the underlying meanings or perspectives that are leading to the organizational behavior. For example, research suggests that teaching hospitals have lower c-section rates than do nonteaching hospitals—but an explanation as to why the organizational behavior developed is not explored. We may speculate that this is the case because teaching hospitals have attending physicians on staff making many of the decisions about women's care and these attending physicians have their malpractice insurance paid by the hospital. In those cases they are not as constrained by the threat of losing that insurance or being responsible for escalating malpractice insurance rates in the case of a lawsuit. But, without speaking to those physicians, this is just speculation.

I suggest that by focusing on what Max Weber calls "explanatory understanding," the puzzle of the c-section epidemic can be solved.[107] Explanatory understanding differs from direct understanding in that explanatory understanding "involves the elucidation of an intervening motivational link between the observed activity and its meaning to the actor."[108] In essence, what is missing from the research on the c-section epidemic is an understanding that is rooted in the *experiences* of maternity care providers and pregnant women. Weber tells us that to understand societal behaviors and trends one must look at the meaningful action of people involved in decisions that lead to those behaviors and trends.[109] According to Randall Collins, a scholar of Weber's work, "to explain something causally is for the analyst to put himself or herself in the place of the actor, to empathically share in his/her worldview and to understand the subjectively meaningful reasons for choosing to act as he/she did."[110] Without subjective understanding, one cannot examine organizational structures, professional norms, and economic and legal incentives when they are actually at the root of many societal trends. Further, without subjective understanding, it becomes easy to blame maternity providers or women for the c-section epidemic, when neither may be responsible for the social processes that set the trend in motion. One must understand the increasing c-section rate from a broader sociological perspective, one that is not present in the medical literature that dominates this discussion and uses in-depth qualitative analysis of maternity providers' and women's experiences to untangle the complex reasons behind the c-section epidemic.

Grounded in an interpretative analysis of the explanatory understanding of social action, I suggest that the increasing c-section rate is a result of the way that health care organizations have responded to their legal and economic environments. To start, it is important to understand that in the United States birth happens almost always in hospitals and that hospitals are organizations with fixed rules to guide individual behavior. I cannot emphasize how important this is. Organizations are abundant in our society, invading every aspect of our lives and often constraining our behavior. Think, for example, of all of the organizations you encounter every day—stores, schools, churches, libraries, hotels, restaurants, hospitals, and the list goes on. We are customers, clients, employees, patients, and members of these organizations, but we are not free to do as we please in them. Our behavior and decisions are greatly constrained by the organizations themselves. Have you ever gone behind the counter at McDonald's to pour your own coffee because the line was too long? Have you nudged the minister aside so that you could deliver a much more rousing sermon or a more sacred blessing? Chances are you have not (or, if you have, you were quickly reprimanded for your actions). You understand the expected rules of behavior in these organizations. Similarly, hospitals are organizations, and maternity providers and pregnant women are expected to understand to behave in certain ways in hospitals. Deviance, or not behaving as expected, has real consequences. Maternity providers may face professional consequences for deviance—for example, being informally scolded by colleagues, formally reprimanded by a supervisor, or having a malpractice insurer deny coverage in the case of a bad outcome. Women also are expected to behave in certain ways. If they do not behave as patients are expected to behave and do what maternity providers ask of them, they may well be defined as "problem patients" and not receive quality care as a result.[111] Maternity providers and women are constrained by hospital rules and expectations for behavior, even if the expected behaviors do not lead to improved outcomes.

This leads me to a discussion of the goals of hospitals. Any organization's goals are complex, and there is no doubt that many employees within hospitals aim to promote the health of individuals. However, another important goal of any organization is survival.[112] Organizations seek to survive into the future, and, to survive, organizations must pay particular attention to their environments, which include customers, suppliers, competitors, and regulatory groups. Organizations must continually assess which parts of the environment are critical to the goal of survival and make sure that they are attending to those aspects. This is the job of organizational managers and administrators.

Let me illustrate this theory by comparing public and private elementary schools. Private schools are much more receptive to input from and demands of individual students and parents than are public schools because private schools are financially dependent on the families' paying tuition. Public schools, on the other hand, are dependent on government for funding, which insulates them from the demands of individual families but causes them to be more focused on meeting state-specified performance criteria on standardized tests, particularly in this era of No-Child-Left-Behind standards. Thus the principals and school boards of private schools are more likely to ask for the input of individual parents in decision making (and ask them for financial contributions) than are public schools.[113] The environmental constraints faced by public and private schools are different, and thus the parts of their environment seen as critical for survival differ.

Hospital administrators also must scan their environment to decide what parts present survival threats. Since the 1980s, hospitals have faced an increasingly competitive economic environment due to changes in Medicare compensation and managed care, both of which have decreased hospital profits.[114] Of particular importance is the change in Medicare compensation. Prior to 1983, Medicare reimbursed hospitals for the costs incurred in treating a patient. That changed with the 1982 Tax Equity and Fiscal Responsibility Act, which stipulated that, beginning in April 1983, Medicare would pay a set fee per case depending on the patient's diagnosis.[115] This move was intended to bring health care costs under control, but it also put hospital profits under competitive pressures because Medicare no longer guaranteed reimbursement of hospital costs.[116] Further, as part of the changes to Medicare reimbursement, the federal government established diagnosis-related groups (DRGs) on which to base payments. The idea was that hospitals would receive a standard payment for each patient with a given diagnosis. This increased standardization in health care with the notion that there is an expected procedure to be done for each diagnosis, which, of course, assumes that all cases falling within a DRG are homogenous.[117]

In response to these economic changes, the health care industry became more consolidated, with the result that large corporations and for-profit hospitals now dominate the delivery of health care in the United States, and these organizations are driven to maximize revenues.[118] Like hospitals overall, big medical practices have grown, and there is striking evidence of the growth of large practices within obstetrics. Between 1996 and 2009, obstetrical practices with more than six physicians increased by 56.3 percent and obstetrical practices with between three and five physicians increased by 9.8 percent, while practices with one or two physicians decreased by 21 percent.[119] The increase of corporatization of medical care and standardization of procedures decreased the autonomy of health care providers.[120] It is interesting to note here that although Medicare does not pay for obstetrics, the corporatization and standardization that DRGs wrought has permeated throughout the entire hospital and is not limited to Medicare cases.

The other significant environmental influence over hospitals has been the legal environment, especially the malpractice insurance market. Hospitals and medical care providers are all subject to complaints of malpractice and, thus, insure against such claims. Malpractice insurance premiums have escalated in recent years, and many obstetricians pay over $100,000 per year for malpractice insurance.[121] Although a physician's probability of being sued has not changed in recent years, a number of multimillion-dollar awards has been seen.[122] In response to these cases and escalating malpractice insurance premiums, the American College of Obstetricians and Gynecologists (ACOG) has declared a "liability crisis" in modern maternity care.[123] From my interviews, physicians are conscious of these legal cases and of escalating malpractice insurance rates, and liability concerns tend to frame their discussions about how birth happens, something I will discuss in chapter 1. In short, health care organizations are embedded in uncertain and competitive economic, political, and legal environments.

As indicated by the growth of large hospitals and practices, organizations do not take uncertainty and threats to survival lying down. Organizations, through the decisions of managers and administrators, respond proactively to uncertain environments in their quest to survive.[124] However, certain organizational contradictions or paradoxes may emerge. For example, changes may occur that contradict organizations' stated goals.[125] Going back to the example of the difference between public and private schools, recall that I suggested public schools are affected by the need to perform well on standardized tests because funding decisions are based on these scores. Within this environment, a scandal broke out in 2011 in the

Washington DC school district, where it was found that forty-one public schools had an unusual number of wrong-answer erasures on a state-mandated standardized test. Wrong answers had been erased and replaced with correct answers; teachers were found to be responsible for the erasures.[126] Although alarming, this should not be particularly surprising because organizational structures had been put in place to link teacher bonuses with improved test scores. Teachers and principals at schools with improved test scores received bonuses as high as $8,000–$10,000. In other words, changes at the organizational level led to contradictions: teachers worked in schools that rewarded them for high-test scores rather than for student learning. A paradox emerged from organizational change—increased test scores did not reflect student learning. The organizational rules not only failed to increase student learning, they also gave teachers (and schools) an incentive to cheat.

Similarly, hospitals, ACOG, and malpractice insurers define liability as a crisis, and with uncertain economic conditions in the health care industry, this crisis has taken on an all-important status. Hospital administrators and risk managers confront this environment and, in response, put in place systems of control to make sure the behavior of individual actors in the organization meets the needs of organizational goals, particularly reducing the liability threat.[127] Thus hospital administrators implement protocols and rules for the use of technology, all of which aim to constrain the behavior of maternity providers to make malpractice claims less likely, but which also contribute to the c-section epidemic. C-section becomes defined as a practice that is the gold standard of care in labor and birth. If a c-section is performed, maternity providers are defined to have done all they can to protect the baby.[128]

Yet these answers to the liability threat produce a contradiction because the c-section epidemic stands in contrast to women's and babies' health, to the economics of health care spending, and, as I'll establish in this book, to the desires of birthing women and health care providers. An organizational paradox has emerged   the c-section epidemic does not protect the health of women or babies or make birth safer or good outcomes more likely. I demonstrate throughout the book how a focus on this epidemic as an organizational paradox created by organizational change helps to explain it.[129] Only by understanding the complex reasons for the escalating c-section rate can we hope to intervene and reverse the trend.

In short, the c-section rate in the United States is the highest in history, and the commonly understood reason for this incredibly high rate is either physician practice or that pregnant women themselves are responsible. Here I suggest that the increasing c-section rate is a result of the way that health care organizations respond to their legal, political, and economic environments. Physicians and women are players within the health care system, but there are many other players who establish the structures, rules, and risks within the organization that constrain physicians and women.

Data

I use several sources of data to study the increasing c-section rate (see the Methods Appendix for complete information). First, I conducted interviews with fifty obstetricians, family physicians who provide maternity care, certified nurse–midwives (CNMs), and labor and delivery nurses in Connecticut, a state that stands out for high c-section and malpractice insurance rates.[130] I gave all maternity providers pseudonyms in the book so that they would feel free to express their views without fear of retribution or exposure of opinions that may be seen as unpopular or inappropriate. The one exception is that I identify Doctor William Barth by name. He was chair of ACOG's Practice Activities Committee at the time of our interview and agreed to speak to me on record as an ACOG representative.

I asked maternity providers to explain why, from their perspective, the c-section rate is increasing. Maternity providers are on the front lines of the increasing c-section rate and offer unparalleled insight into reasons for the escalation. I was surprised at the uncompensated time providers gave to me—sometimes over two hours—and the eagerness with which some sought me out. I often arrived at my office to find voice mail messages from maternity providers who wanted to be interviewed. They have stories to tell, and their perception is that no one is listening. I listened and have incorporated their insights into this book. Maternity providers know the c-section rate is being influenced by nonmedical factors, yet they are, understandably, reluctant to publicly admit that their decisions may be influenced by factors not related to the health of women and babies.

It may seem that the type of maternity provider (i.e., physician, midwife, nurse) is interchangeable at times. In fact, I find that, most times, providers think in very similar ways about modern maternity care because they are all actors within hospitals. Even so, maternity providers are affected differently by the systems of control put in place by organizations to oversee their behavior. Thus, at times, you will also see how, although all types of maternity providers often talk similarly about the constraints they face, because they are affected by the systems of control in different ways, nurses, midwives, and physicians sometimes have different experiences. For example, nurses typically feel more bound by hospital protocols than do physicians because the hospital employs nurses and provides their malpractice insurance. Nurses tell me that the hospital will "hang them out to dry" if they do not follow protocol and something goes wrong, even if the bad outcome is not the result of a breech in protocol.

Second, my research team conducted interviews with eighty-three postpartum women at a Connecticut hospital. We interviewed all women the day after they gave birth. Women's experiences are integral to this discussion. Throughout the book, I use women's stories to understand how women think about, plan for, and experience birth. We did not record the names of the women interviewed, and the names used throughout the book are fictitious; again, we did this so that they would feel free to express their views without fear of retribution or concern that they would be seen as problem patients if they relayed to us a negative birth experience. We also made very clear to the women that we were independent researchers and not hospital employees.

I use *Cochrane Collaboration Reviews* as the source for information on evidence-based obstetrical practice. Cochrane is a nonprofit, independent, international organization established in 1988 to disseminate evidence-based and systematic reviews of medical interventions.[131] When Cochrane has not reviewed a procedure, I summarize the existing empirical literature on the topic. In terms of empirical evidence on national trends of women's experiences, I draw on three quantitative studies: Listening to Mothers II (LTMII), a national survey conducted in the United States of women who gave birth in 2005; the Centers for Disease Control's (CDC) Births: Final Data for 2010, the most recent analysis of birth trends in the United States; and Births: Preliminary Data for 2011, which has the most recent data on a limited number of measures.[132]

Organization of the Book

In the first part of the book I examine the liability environment of obstetrical care. In chapter 1, I describe the liability environment faced by maternity providers and also their subjective understanding of that environment.

The second part of the book examines how the control systems that constrain the actions and decisions of maternity providers have been implemented in hospitals to reduce liability threats. I argue they have also contributed to the increasing c-section rate. In chapter 2 I examine protocols and the patient safety movement. I suggest that liability concerns have shaped protocol changes as much, if not more, than safety concerns and that an increasing c-section rate is part and parcel of the dominant patient safety movement in obstetrics. In chapter 3 I go on to examine technologies used in labor and birth and show that most are not supported by empirical evidence that they improve birth outcomes. Rather, they are used to protect maternity providers from the blame of a bad outcome and to carefully control a woman's labor and birth. The result is more and more c-sections.

In the third part of the book I show how organizational constraints affect repeat c-sections and women's choices. In chapter 4 I examine how liability concerns lead to the practice of repeat c-sections. Vaginal birth after c-section (VBAC) rarely happens in the modern United States because organizations take away this option for many women *and* maternity providers. Chapter 5 looks at how women's choices are restrained in modern maternity care by organizational constraints. Finally, in the conclusion, I end the book by looking at how to address the epidemic c-section rate with rational change. I suggest specific solutions to bring the tide of increasing c-sections under control.

My hope in writing this book is that the high percentage of c-section births in the United States will be publicly recognized as an epidemic threatening the wellbeing of women, babies, and families. With this recognition, we can begin to insist that current practices in hospitals be changed so that women and maternity providers can do what they know (and science shows) is best—to promote vaginal birth. At the very least, a wide-reaching conversation needs to be started with open, honest communication among all parties involved.

PART I

The Root of the Problem

1

The Liability Threat in Obstetrics

When I was a resident, I had a very old Chair who said something that stuck with me [and] helps me explain where we are now. . . . He said that he's never done a cesarean that he regretted. He had done dozens and dozens of vaginal deliveries that he did, but never a cesarean. And I think that is where doctors are right now. . . . You're unlikely to be the person who does the next section and gets surgical complications, but you could be the one regretting that vaginal delivery if the baby doesn't come out perfect.

—Physician Jacob Chism

Doctor Chism, an obstetrician of twelve years at the time of the interview, is quite frank about his concern with being blamed for a bad vaginal birth outcome. His is not alone in this concern. The American College of Obstetricians and Gynecologists (ACOG), the professional association representing most obstetricians and gynecologists in the United States, has named malpractice liability a crisis for the profession and physicians' practice of defensive medicine a consequence. In a September 11, 2009 press release announcing findings from a survey of its members about professional liability, Albert L. Strunk, ACOG Deputy Executive Vice President, stated, "The latest survey shows that the medical liability situation for ob-gyns remains a *chronic crisis* and continues to deprive women of all ages—especially pregnant women—of experienced ob-gyns. Women's health care suffers as ob-gyns further decrease obstetric services, reduce gynecologic procedures, and are *forced to practice defensive medicine*."[1] In other words, ACOG suggests that physicians practice defensively to avoid lawsuits—this is code for performing more c-sections.

The Legal Environment of Obstetrics

As discussed earlier, the legal environment of health care has gone through rapid changes. To understand these changes, it is important to understand the role of insurance cycles. All types of insurance are known to go through cycles. "Hard cycles" are characterized by a lack of insurance policies and high prices, while "soft cycles" are characterized by a good supply of policies, a lack of demand, and low prices. Thinking specifically about the market for malpractice insurance, physicians and hospitals feel the pinch in hard markets because malpractice insurance policies are expensive and sometimes hard to find.[2] Defined hard markets in the malpractice insurance industry have happened in the United States during 1975–78, 1984–87, and 2001–4.[3] Maternity providers and ACOG describe these as periods of "malpractice crisis." Notice that the hard cycles are relatively common and last for about three years. Although experts suggest that the most recent hard cycle in the malpractice insurance industry ended in 2004, it is not clear from talking with maternity providers or following statements from ACOG that they believe it has.

Obstetrics is notably one of the fields of medicine most affected by these cycles and has the added problem that malpractice claims are infrequent, large, and hard to predict, all of which contribute to uncertainty.[4] For obstetrical medical malpractice claims opened or closed during the period January 1, 2009, through December 31, 2011, the most common primary allegation of the claims was neurological impairment (28.8 percent) and stillbirth or neonatal death (14.4 percent).[5] The most common neurological impairment cases are for shoulder dystocia (where the baby's shoulders unpredictably get stuck behind the woman's pubic bone) and cerebral palsy (a disability involving the central nervous system that is largely believed to be due to something that occurs during a woman's pregnancy). Incidents of shoulder dystocia and cerebral palsy are notably difficult to predict or prevent, and thus maternity providers feel that most negative birth outcomes involving shoulder dystocia or cerebral palsy are due to obstetrical maloccurrence, defined as "a bad or undesirable outcome that is *unrelated to the quality of care provided*," rather than to obstetrical malpractice, which is defined as "a bad or undesirable outcome *caused by medical negligence*."[6] However, maternity providers believe that they will be held responsible for such birth outcomes regardless of whether they committed a medical error.

It can be argued that because most obstetrical lawsuits are tied to hard-to-predict events (shoulder dystocia and cerebral palsy) and may even occur before labor begins (cerebral palsy), the type of malpractice risk maternity providers face is markedly different from that in other medical specialties. Some births will have perfect outcomes, while others will involve birth defects and death regardless of the care a woman receives during labor and birth. Thus, one can see the precarious problem maternity providers face. This is not to say that malpractice in maternity care does not happen. Certainly there are documented cases of substandard care where women and babies are harmed because of the type or quality of care or lack of care they receive.[7] But the malpractice risk is quite different for maternity providers compared to other medical providers, and they feel this difference.

From the obstetrician's perspective, the risk of lawsuit is real. In a 2012 ACOG survey, 77.3 percent of responding obstetricians reported having had at least one lawsuit filed against them in their career, with an average of 2.69 lawsuits per obstetrician.[8] In fact, nearly every physician in high-risk specialties, including obstetrics, will be subject to a malpractice claim by the age of sixty-five.[9] While obstetricians have the third-highest rate of suit after neurologists and neurosurgeons, the average claim payment for obstetricians is almost 20 percent higher than the overall average claim payment for all specialties, and obstetricians have the highest total number of claims paid among all medical specialties.[10] The average claim payment for ob-gyns in 2012 was $510,473 and differs markedly by primary allegation: $982,051 for neurological impairment; $364,794 for "other infant injury—major"; and $271,149 for stillbirth or neonatal death.[11]

In terms of the disposition of malpractice claims, examining claims closed between January 1, 2009, and December 31, 2011, 43.9 percent were dropped by plaintiffs' attorneys or were settled with no payment to the plaintiff, 38.7 percent were settled by a payment to the plaintiff on behalf of the obstetrician, and 17.4 percent were closed through a jury or court verdict or through arbitration.[12] When the lawsuit went to trial, the court decided in favor of the obstetrician in 65.6 percent of those cases.[13] Doing some quick math, what this means is that payment on behalf of the obstetrician (either through settlement or court verdict) happens in less than half (44.7 percent) of malpractice cases.

These contradictory trends—a high risk of being sued but a smaller risk that the suit will result in a payment to the plaintiff—sometimes lead critics to question the existence of a malpractice crisis.[14] Other conflicting trends also lead to this doubt. For example, the *number* of obstetrical malpractice claims is *not* increasing and has actually decreased in the United States generally and in Connecticut specifically over the past twenty-five years (see figure 1.1).[15] But the average *payment* in malpractice suits are increasing nationally and in Connecticut (see figure 1.2). In the United States malpractice claim payouts increased from an average of $254,019 in 1991 to $330,435 in 2010 (in 2010 dollars), a 30 percent increase.[16] The average payment on a malpractice claim in Connecticut increased by slightly more, 38 percent, in the same period, from $314,206 in 1991 to $433,446 in 2010 (in constant 2010 dollars), although this average hides spikes in this measure, including an average of $817,092 in 2008.[17]

Malpractice insurance rates are also high and increasing at record rates nationally and in Connecticut. The average cost of policies offered to obstetricians by malpractice insurance companies in Connecticut increased by 92 percent from $73,451 in 1997 to $140,902 in 2012 (in constant 2012 dollars).[18] Although harder to document because of regional variation, obstetrical malpractice rates have also increased nationally. For example, by one measure malpractice rates increased by 70 percent between 2000 and 2004.[19]

Connecticut has other characteristics that make it an interesting state to study. A 2009 report from the State of Connecticut Insurance Department concluded that Connecticut has the highest annual cost per malpractice claim.[20] Further, Connecticut has had three record-breaking obstetrical malpractice awards in the past several years: in 2005 a $36.5 million cerebral palsy award; in 2008 a $38.5 million award for a neurologically impaired infant; and in 2011 a $58.6 million cerebral palsy award. The 2011 $58.6 million award replaced the 2008 $38.5 million award as the largest medical malpractice award in Connecticut history.[21] Connecticut also does not have a cap on noneconomic damages, commonly referred to as a tort-cap, which is something ACOG stresses as a cure for liability crisis.

At the same time that the liability threat has been emphasized for maternity providers, changes in malpractice insurance coverage have caused them increased uncertainty. To deal with the risk of malpractice suits, maternity providers carry malpractice insurance; in fact, they are usually mandated by hospitals to purchase malpractice insurance to protect themselves in malpractice claims. There are two types of malpractice insurance: occurrence policies and claims-made policies. Occurrence policies cover all incidents that occur in the year the insurance premium is paid, regardless of when the claim is filed.[22] For example, if a baby was born in 2008

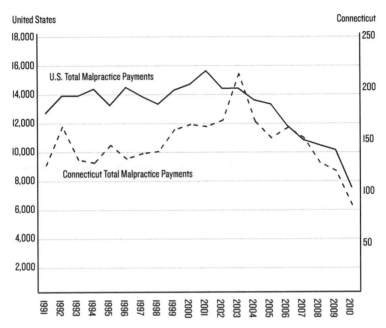

Figure 1.1. Number of Malpractice Payments in the U.S. and Connecticut, 1991–2010.

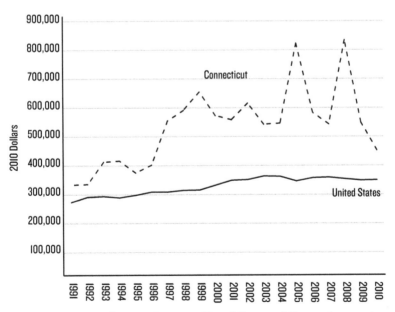

Figure 1.2. Average Malpractice Payments, United States and Connecticut, 1996–2010, in 2010 Dollars.

and her parents file a malpractice claim in 2012, the physician's malpractice insurance premiums paid in 2008 will cover him or her for that claim. This is in contrast to claims-made policies, which covers claims *filed* during the year the insurance premium is paid.[23] In this same example, the physician's 2008 premiums would cover only claims *filed* by a patient in 2008, meaning that if a birth occurred in 2008 and a claim of malpractice is filed in 2012, the 2012 premium would cover the claim.

The malpractice insurance industry has increasingly shifted to offering physicians claims-made policies. For example, in 2012, 61.6 percent of obstetricians had claims-made policies, while only 30.3 percent had occurrence coverage (8.1 percent of obstetricians were self-insured or had another unidentified type of malpractice insurance).[24] Claims-made policies are advantageous to medical malpractice insurance companies because these policies decrease the length of time between policy payment and settlement.[25] Insurers prefer shorter lags between policy payment and claims payment because there is less of a chance that inflation will have an effect on the size of the settlement or that a precedent-setting case will be decided that will increase the likelihood of a family winning a malpractice case.[26]

However, this shift in insurance coverage has had deleterious effects on physicians, "trapping" them in the profession because if they retire or stop practicing obstetrics they must still pay malpractice insurance premiums to cover any future claims that may be filed within the medical malpractice statute of limitations, which varies by state, but is on average twelve years for newborns.[27] To stop obstetrical practice, physicians must pay a hefty "tail insurance" premium—typically 1.5 to 2 times the annual premium—that covers claims filed after the year the last premium was paid through the last year a patient could file a medical malpractice claim under the current statute of limitations.[28] This disadvantage was noted by a number of obstetricians, one of whom, Rosemary Steel, a relatively young obstetrician in her mid-thirties, is already aware of this issue: "Most malpractice insurance carriers will give claims-made insurance coverage. . . . [I am] only covered for the time that [I am] around paying the bill, and then, if I want to move away, I need to pay a tail. . . . So, I'm kind of shackled to where I am."

Maternity Providers' Understanding of the Liability Environment

This feeling of being shackled because of changes in malpractice insurance policies is just the start of how aware maternity providers are of liability risk. Let me share a story to illustrate. I plan to drive across the state to interview physician Philip Burgin, but my schedule becomes too cluttered to manage the drive. I e-mail Doctor Burgin and offer to interview him by phone. I am surprised when he offers to make the three-hour round trip so that we can meet in person. Of course I agree, wondering why he is going to this trouble. We meet over coffee at a community college near my home, and it quickly becomes clear that Doctor Burgin is on a mission—to tell about the fear, anxiety, and worry he faces on a daily basis as an obstetrician. The meeting starts out as a lecture, but he softens once he figures out that I came not to indict him but rather to understand from his perspective why the c-section rate is increasing. What I learn from him is that every day he thinks about being sued and worries about not being able to put his children through college because he might lose his ability to practice. "Do you face those fears as a college professor?" he asks me.

The fear and anxiety over liability expressed by Doctor Burgin are near-ubiquitous concerns expressed by the maternity providers I interviewed. Their anxiety and fear are tied to several potential professional and economic outcomes that might result from being named in a malpractice lawsuit, outcomes from which malpractice insurance does not protect them. I have grouped these anxieties into five themes.

The first anxiety is that if a maternity provider is involved in a malpractice suit, he or she may lose malpractice insurance coverage and subsequently face escalating malpractice insurance premiums. Physician Tony Oday says, "I know somebody recently who lost her insurance because she had three lawsuits. . . . She's a good physician. She just had some bad luck." Likewise, physician Leticia Stites worries that "if you have a case and you lose, you lose your ability to practice because your rates go so high you can't afford it." These two fears—being dropped from coverage and facing high premiums—go hand in hand. Malpractice insurance companies do not raise the premiums of high-risk physicians; these companies rarely "experience rate" medical providers.[29] What this means is that malpractice insurance companies charge the same premium to all obstetricians. Thus, rather than increasing the insurance rates of obstetricians who have malpractice claims filed against them, malpractice insurers may cancel their policies.[30] In such a case the provider will have to obtain malpractice insurance from a surplus line carrier, "insurers who specialize in hard-to-insure risks," and likely pay a much higher premium.[31]

A second anxiety is that a settlement or award will exceed a provider's malpractice insurance cap, usually $1 million, and that his or her personal assets will be vulnerable. Physician Lois Timberlake articulates this fear: "I think we've all heard about these cases, where it's $15 million, $20 million [awards]. . . . You have limits on your policy, and if the award is beyond your limits, they can go after your house, your car, your whatever, which is a very scary thought." This concern is not without reason. A study of medical malpractice claims between 1991 and 2005 found that obstetricians were the most likely of physicians in all medical specialties to have claims closed in excess of $1 million.[32]

A third anxiety deals with the actual process of the lawsuit and the time and effort it takes to be involved in a malpractice proceeding. Nurse Jane Rios describes how this anxiety affects physicians:

> We've had . . . physicians [who] have gone through [a lawsuit], and they've actually won their cases. But the time, the effort, the gray hairs that lead up to that day that you actually win the case—you age yourself ten to fifteen years just with all the stuff that you have to go through to get to it. And, yes, you win [but] . . . you would never want to do [it] again.

Part of the frustration mentioned by Nurse Rios is no doubt due to the length of time it takes to resolve claims of medical malpractice. Between 1999 and 2002 the average length of time from the occurrence of an alleged malpractice to the closing of the malpractice claim in obstetrics was four years, but 13 percent of claims took seven or more years from occurrence to resolution.[33] Physician Philip Burgin pinpoints this anxiety when he tells me, "Being in a suit is a nightmare. It totally envelops your life for the five to seven years it takes to play out. You're constantly worried; you're constantly doubting yourself; you have nervous anxiety attacks; you have acid stomach. . . . Imagine the worst thing [that] can happen hanging over your head for seven years."

Beyond economic fears of paying high malpractice premiums or losing personal assets in a lawsuit, maternity providers worry about their reputations being impinged by being publicly exposed as having committed malpractice. Physician Joe Haley greets me in the lobby of the hospital. "Can I buy you coffee?" he asks. Fresh coffee in hand, we ride the elevator to the labor and delivery floor—he is on call today—and search for an empty seminar room. On our way he greets nurses by name with a smile and a wave. He is friendly and seems quite popular. We find a seminar room and sit down across the table from each other. He slides a few sheets of paper in front of me. He has printed out material from prosecuting malpractice attorneys' websites about obstetrical malpractice suits they have won and points out to me how they negatively portray the physician involved. He points me to one about a friend of his who was sued: "You're named on a public website [reading from the printout]: 'If the evidence had shown that [City] Hospital and Dr. [Jager] [his friend] were not at fault, we would have gone that way. We didn't see anything that showed us remotely that they weren't liable.'" Physician Haley was particularly disturbed by this case because, knowing the details, he felt that Dr. Jager had not committed a medical error.

Finally, maternity providers worry that a lawsuit will haunt them for the rest of their professional careers. Physician Geneva Spalding tells me, "Once you've been named in a suit, forever and ever . . . every time you apply for licensing . . . you have to write a whole paragraph about the [incident]. . . . It follows you. . . . If you move to another state, you need to get a certificate from the state." Midwife Rita Morey concurs with this frustration: "Once you have had a suit brought against you, regardless of the outcome, when you go to get privileged at any institution, you have to report it, and you have to explain what happened, why you were sued, what the outcome was, and why. And it becomes a really onerous process."

Being involved with a negative birth outcome exacerbates these anxieties. Physician Joe Haley tells me that after a negative birth outcome, "you look at the mailbox every day if you have an outcome like [shoulder dystocia], and you're going to see the return address from some sort of litigator's firm. And you watch the mailbox every day. It's really painful." It is clear from my conversation with him that Doctor Haley is consumed with anxiety, much of which is due to his being personally involved in a malpractice case.

Physician Andrew Robinette, another physician I interview in the hospital while he is on call, has a similar take on what it is like to be sued:

> The stress on family, on marriages, on sense of self-esteem. . . . There are better ways to make money than being an obstetrician   be an orthopedist, be a radiologist. . . . But people do this essentially because they really want to help people. And you get sued. . . . In cases that these often arise from, they are frantically trying to do their best. It's a situation of high stress where you've got to make on-the-spot decisions. . . . Their adrenaline is high; they're emotionally invested, and, yet, things don't go well. And then you get sued for it. . . . You're beating yourself up already. Can you imagine what that does to someone's self-esteem?

What was clear to me in talking with maternity providers and is so eloquently stated by Doctor Robinette is that maternity providers typically go into maternity care because they want to help women and babies. They fear bad outcomes not just because they'll be sued, but also because they want to promote the health of women and babies. The anxiety they face is that they will be held responsible for bad outcomes that they tried their absolute hardest to prevent. This is a common notion expressed by maternity providers. Physician Terri Diggs sums this up nicely:

> With obstetrics there is so much unpredictability, and bad things that can occur despite the most optimal care given. . . . It's likely that the doctor will be sued whether or not they did anything wrong. . . . You have a jury that feels sympathetic to a damaged infant. They want to blame somebody, and they tend to blame the doctor, even if it has nothing to do with the care given by the doctor.

Doctor Diggs sees obstetrics as a special case, and most maternity providers feel this way. They feel that the unpredictability of bad birth outcomes means that these unfortunate occurrences are random events, though ones for which the doctors are held responsible. In fact, the academic literature on the malpractice supports this fear. For example, most malpractice payments are awarded for injuries that are not the result of medical error.[34] Further, research also finds that physicians who have had malpractice suits are not necessarily providing worse care than those who have not had suits.[35] This fear of the randomness of lawsuits is captured in the following interview excerpt from physician Leticia Stites:

> Most people have had lawsuits either discussed or papers served for a lawsuit, and I think it's random. It's like "ticktock." It's just going to happen to you one day because, again, it has nothing to do with how you practice, whether you're good or bad, whether malpractice has occurred or not, it just happens.

This feeling that obstetrical outcomes are not predictable and are not due to medical error is also apparent in way that physicians describe lawsuits. An example that came up repeatedly in my interviews is that of a severely disabled child. Physicians feel that monetary settlement happens in these cases regardless of whether medical error was committed. Research suggests that they have a point. The severity of a disability, rather than negligence, best predicts the payment of claims.[36] The following interview excerpt serves as an example of how physicians talk about being blamed for outcomes over which they feel they have no control. Notice in the following excerpt how physician Robert Hinson frames himself as a victim of the current malpractice legal environment, a common sentiment among obstetricians:

> I got sued for being a Good Samaritan once. . . . I got sued for a baby that had six feet of umbilical cord around the neck and a knot in that umbilical [cord]. And I delivered that baby by cesarean section. And that baby was not good neurologically thereafter. . . . And I settled that case because my [family member], who is an attorney, said to me, "If you take that baby and put it in front of the jury, they're not going to listen to anything that you have to say, and they're going to look at the baby and say, 'You're the deep pocket. We're going to give them more money than what you would have settled for,'" which was millions of dollars.

Another way physicians expressed this frustration of being held accountable for things beyond their control is how cases are sometimes settled on their behalf, because settling a case means admitting medical error. Physician Maggie Rust tells me, "We don't necessarily like that the hospital settles because then they're kind of admitting fault. And then . . . we get a little defensive: 'We didn't do anything wrong. Don't settle with them.' But we do understand that it's cheaper sometimes for them to settle. But it is, it's frustrating either way." Notice again the articulation of a feeling of a loss of control.

It should also be understood that physicians are not the only ones who worry about being sued. Nurses and midwives share the fear that they will be held accountable for unpredictable outcomes. For example, nurses talk about the stress of dealing with patients who write down everything that happens during labor and birth and tell the nurses they will sue for any negative outcome. Nurse April Coleman describes this: "It's unbelievable how people come in looking for trouble. [They] tell you right off that they're keeping an eye on everything you do. . . . They're very forward about it . . . 'You better do everything right or I'm going to sue you.'"

I also heard of patients talking with providers at prenatal and well checkups about malpractice cases they know about from the news:

> People will come in and tell you these stories about how stupid this provider was and killed this baby, . . . and they clearly don't have . . . the clinical

information to even know what really happened in the situation. . . . You have to be very careful because what they've said about other providers, goodness, they can be saying that about you if something bad happened.

Midwife Crystal Hereford is clear in her interview that liability is often on her mind. Similarly, nurse Anne Boudreaux shares this story with me: "When I worked at [City Hospital], I think that every nurse [who] worked there had been depositioned [in a malpractice case]. Every one. They were all talking about it all the time, [saying], 'Well, we have to do that because, what if we got sued?'"

I Wish I Hadn't Gone into This Field

Maternity providers' anxiety about liability has a number of consequences, one of which is a common regret about having gone into the obstetrics profession. For example, physician Joe Haley tells me that he discouraged his own children from entering a medical profession and was relieved when they went down different career paths. He did not want them to experience the anxiety he feels on a daily basis, an anxiety he believes is unavoidable in the medical world, especially obstetrics. Physicians expressed regret regularly about their own choice of occupation. Physician Janice O'Brien relays an interesting experience in which she and other obstetricians were attempting to recruit medical students into their specialty:

> The American College of Ob-Gyn [ACOG] put out a big effort to . . . recruit people to our [specialty], and we had meetings with the students at Yale and [University of Connecticut]. . . . And it was hard because all the guys in practice are trying to say this is a great profession . . . and yet we're all going, "I [would not] to do it again."

She described their disingenuousness in their recruitment efforts because they recognized they would not choose this profession if they had it to do over again. They had regrets.

Beyond having negative feelings about the profession, some physicians drop out of obstetrical practice altogether. I interviewed two gynecologists who had recently stopped practicing obstetrics and heard tales of others who had done the same—one who is now "home baking cookies." Gynecologist Terri Diggs tells me of her decision: "The fear of litigation especially in regards to obstetrics is just profound in this state and the cost both financially and emotionally I just thought were in excess of what I was willing [to pay] to continue doing OB." Doctor Diggs is not alone in her analysis. Survey research finds that physicians with high malpractice insurance rates are less satisfied with their careers, and physicians often cite liability risk as the reason they stop practicing obstetrics.[37] Midwives and nurses also experience a desire to leave the profession to avoid liability threats. One nurse I interviewed is working on her credentials to become a nurse–practitioner, a job she thinks will be less stressful than being a labor and delivery nurse. Another nurse squelched her hopes of becoming a midwife because she did not want to increase her liability risk. Similarly, midwife Ada Medlin speaks about her dilemma with continuing obstetrical care: "There were some recent suits in the state [involving] . . . midwives [who] I knew very well, and who are great, wonderful providers, and it just makes you kind of think twice. . . . Do I want to take this risk? Is it worth it with a family, at this point in my life, to do this?"

Practicing Defensively: A Way to Survive

Another way maternity providers deal with liability anxiety is to practice defensively. It is common to hear that physicians practice "defensive medicine"—that is, they perform procedures and tests not to protect the health of the patient but rather to prevent malpractice liability. From my interviews, it is clear this is not just conjecture in the case of obstetrics. Defensive practices happen regularly. For example, physician Jack Bianco tells me:

> I will promise you a third of what I do is defensive medicine . . . if you really want to use honest criteria. Do I really believe I have to do everything that I do? No. But I do it because if something bad happens, someone can't blame me for not having done it. . . . Am I causing harm by doing a c-section in this situation? I potentially am. But I can't control that.

Renowned political theorist Carl J. Friedrich refers to such defensive practices as "the rule of anticipated reaction."[38] This concept refers to authoritative structures that guide individuals on how to act to avoid negative consequences or to secure positive consequences. In the context of c-sections, the rule of anticipated reaction operates when a physician decides to perform a c-section or other interventions because of a belief that he or she will be less likely to be sued for doing the surgery than for facilitating a vaginal birth. It is important to understand, however, that as much as the public responds negatively to the term "defensive medicine," individual maternity providers do not decide on the action that is defensive. Rather, defensive practices are defined by organizations as a way to prevent liability, in this case c-sections. Such a definition has authority over providers, even though it may not be obvious that organizations have this type of control. I argue here that organizations such as ACOG, malpractice insurers, courts, and hospitals have defined liability as a problem and c-sections as the solution to this problem. Practicing defensively takes a number of forms.

Document Everything: The Best Solution in the Case of a Bad Outcome

A common response to liability anxiety of maternity providers—nurses, midwives, and physicians—is a heightened focus on documentation. Documentation becomes a way for maternity providers to demonstrate that they are providing adequate care; they have learned that *lack of documentation* may be used in a malpractice claim to suggest that a bad outcome was due to medical error. Maternity providers must constantly document that they did the right thing. If something isn't documented, it's as good as not done. Especially because of the unpredictable nature of many adverse obstetrical outcomes, a focus on documentation of every labor and every birth becomes almost obsessive among providers. They don't know which labor will end badly. This means every case has to be well documented. Below are two telling examples of how maternity providers use increased vigilance in documentation to avert liability threats:

> I think about malpractice with every single patient I encounter, . . . and the doctor who doesn't is asking for trouble. . . .Every phone call, every office visit, every hospital encounter—I think about malpractice. . . . Every time I write a note about a phone call, about an office visit, or about something else in the hospital, I think, "How will this look in court?" (Physician Philip Burgin)

I'm always thinking, "Am I going to be able to stand up in court with what I'm writing? . . . Is this going to pass muster if I'm on the stand?" You always have to keep that in mind as you're doing your documentation. (Nurse April Colman)

Nurses face a particular burden of documentation because unlike most physicians—who are typically self-employed or employed by obstetrical practices—nurses are almost always employed by hospitals, and hospitals provide malpractice insurance for their employees. The hitch, however, is that hospitals will not cover a nurse in a malpractice claim if she did not document that protocols were followed. In fact, consistently breaking protocols is a cause for termination of employment. As nurse Michele Saxton tells me, "If you're not keeping up on your reading and you're not up on your standards of care and you don't know the protocols, you'll get yourself in trouble. They won't protect you if you didn't follow those procedural policies." Thus nurses become the "enforcers" of protocols; the burden of "compliance" is placed on the least-powerful professional actors, a common practice in organizations. This burden was a common concern of nurses. Some may be surprised to hear that most nurses with whom I spoke are very critical of the way maternity care is being delivered, with a particular scorn toward interventions, such as routine inductions, use of Pitocin for labor acceleration, and, especially, nonmedically indicated c-sections. I think this would especially surprise many midwives, who often have a somewhat cynical view of nurses. Nurses are structurally placed in a situation where they must enforce protocols and document that those protocols have been followed.

Excessive documentation becomes a common practice, and this imperative is spread throughout the profession in conferences and workshops that focus on malpractice prevention. These conferences and workshops almost inevitably emphasize the importance of documentation. Doctor Burgin follows up our interview with an e-mail message about a conference that teaches the importance of documentation to prevent liability:

I thought it might interest you to know that I am going to a full-day seminar entitled: "Advanced Fetal Monitoring 2007 and Legal Implications." There's no mistaking what this course is about. One of the lectures is titled: "Monitoring for Asphyxia: What You Need to Know and *Document.*" The reality of the event is the same, but how you document it (and therefore how it's presented to a jury) is what counts. I think about law all day long.

Conferences spread documentation as the answer to liability threat and also perpetuate a focus on law among maternity providers.

Nurses and midwives attend the same type of conference presentations on malpractice prevention, as this interview excerpt from labor and delivery nurse Margie Napolitano suggests: "Definitely in the past five years or so, it's become a lot more scary for nurses and doctors because of the lawsuits and the legal issues. And a lot of conferences are focused on legal issues and documentation and all that." Midwives also discuss these types of conferences and presentations; for example, midwife Rosalie Batten describes how "in [university] teaching hospitals we have a risk reduction program. . . . We have to do this continuing-ed piece specifically for the insurance company for the risk-reduction program. . . . So we are constantly being bombarded with, 'This is the best legal defense.'"

C-Sections: They're Just Less Risky for Us

One can see how, put in such a position, maternity providers may focus too much on how attorneys will perceive their actions. For example, physician Philip Burgin tells me, "[I think], 'This wouldn't have been a shoulder dystocia if you hadn't delivered that head.' Because the question posed to a doctor [is], 'If you'd done a c-section, would this baby be paralyzed now?' I hear lawyers talking in my head all the time." It is clear that Doctor Burgin thinks about liability and how attorneys will interpret his actions constantly, likely obsessively.

I heard tales of maternity providers' observing deviations from a normal labor and dwelling on similarities to previous bad outcomes, another defensive practice. This tendency is described well by midwife Crystal Hereford: "I can just think of so many physicians, [when] I'd have somebody in labor, . . . [the] physician saying, 'She has twenty minutes more, and I'm doing the c-section, because all I can think about is that last bad outcome I had.'"

Imagining bad outcomes and lawyers talking in their heads is just a short step to intervening any time labor is not going according to plan. As Physician Leticia Stites tells me, "That's where the scariness comes in. That it can be no fault of your own, an act of God, or just a spontaneous event, and you still get sued, and you still lose. So, here you have no control over that situation and . . . it definitely leads to a higher c-section rate where the outcome is immediate, and it's controlled, and no one can blame you for it." Similarly, physician Philip Burgin said, "I think if we do more c-sections it is going to result in [fewer] lawsuits. Not because there will be less difficult babies. I think we're still going to have cerebral palsy because no one knows what causes it. But because if you do a c-section you've done all you can do. Now the only question is did you do it early enough."

This easing into c-sections as a solution to liability threats becomes more apparent after a maternity provider is sued for malpractice. The threshold to move to a surgical delivery slips lower and lower. Many physicians reported to me that after they had been sued they began to jump more quickly to performing a c-section, another example of Friedrich's rule of anticipated action.[39] They are performing c-sections because they have learned that doing so may prevent a malpractice lawsuit. The following two interview excerpts illustrate this:

> It became more personal when I was sued. . . . There was particularly one case . . . I don't know if the child would have been OK or not. But that was the allegation—that a c-section would have helped. . . . After that my threshold became much lower. Although probably 95, 99 percent of the patients with that same situation would have been OK, I kept thinking to myself, "OK, for that one percent, it's such a catastrophic outcome for the child, for the parents, and then for me, not only because I care for the patient, but then going through the whole process of a suit." . . . Nobody really wants to take that chance. And so you don't. (Physician Lois Timberlake)

> I have been [what] I'll call the victim of medical malpractice lawsuits, and with that experience and also . . . now paying over $120,000 a year for malpractice premiums, I've realized that there's a huge implication of our legal system on why the cesarean section rates are going up. And, I think, if I were to move tomorrow to Montreal [Canada] and practice medicine, my cesarean section rate would immediately go down because I would not be set up in the same manner of really intimidation by what's happening out there. (Physician Robert Hinson)[40]

Nurses also see physicians jumping quickly to c-sections, especially after a physician has been involved in a malpractice suit. Nurse Amanda Barnett tells me:

You watch how the physicians are practicing now, and because of malpractice and things that have happened in our own state. . . . Doctors [who] I have worked with for fourteen years, who we call the men and women with "all the feel," they would watch a strip [with] variables and decels, and they'd [say], "Let's try this, let's try that—change position, use amnioinfusion, give herb tea," whatever. . . . Let's just say there were five things that you could do when a strip looked bad. Now they are trying one or two things, and if it's not immediately better, we go down the hall for a c-section.

Perhaps the most shocking story I heard comes from physician Joe Haley, the mild-mannered, friendly obstetrician who bought me coffee. He lowers his eyes and speaks quietly when he says, "I call my wife when I'm hanging out in labor and delivery, and I say, 'Oh, the strip looks like this,' and she says, 'Just do a section.' [I feel threatened], and in a serious way, because . . . I mean, she's not a doctor. But you really are vulnerable, and there's really no protection." This is perhaps the most telling example of the fear maternity providers face in modern maternity care. Asking one's nonphysician spouse for advice on how to manage a woman's labor seems unbelievable, but it does happen, perhaps in this case as a way Doctor Haley manages his stress and anxiety over caring for women with complicated deliveries.

Where the Authoritative Rules Originate: The Role of Organizations

Maternity providers feel caught in a bind. The defined way to escape being held accountable for unpreventable negative birth outcomes is to perform a c-section. Then, if a bad outcome happens, they are less likely to be blamed—they did all they could. From the perspective of maternity providers, they are caught in the fundamental irrationality of organizational change. Organizations have defined c-sections as the answer to liability threat. This definition causes maternity providers to change their behavior and perform more c-sections because they fear if they do not they will be blamed for bad birth outcomes, even those outcomes that are not preventable or predictable. The current economic, political, and legal environment binds organizations, and organizations change to protect organizational interests. In this case, professional organizations, malpractice insurers, courts, and hospitals have coalesced in their suggestion that c-sections solve liability threats.

The most common way that providers learn about c-sections being a solution to liability is by being involved in a lawsuit or hearing about a malpractice lawsuit where the maternity provider is asked by the litigating attorney why a c-section was not performed, with the underlying accusation being that a c-section would have prevented the bad outcome. Physician Lawrence Rascon makes clear his feeling that courts have defined c-sections as the solution to bad birth outcomes and liability threats:

> Every time an obstetrician gets sued for a bad outcome of a pregnancy, the one thing in every trial is, "You should have done the cesarean section." . . . And I think you hear that every single time and every malpractice case you hear or read about: . . . "You should have done a section," or "You should have done a section earlier." . . . And after a while everybody says, "Well, if that's what we have to do, then that's what we have to do."

Courts also enforce this view by focusing on the timing of the c-section. For example, physician Robert Hinson tells me, "When you get deposed in a malpractice lawsuit . . . you will be asked if you could have done the cesarean five or ten minutes earlier or done it an hour earlier . . . and could that have made the difference." In short, what maternity providers tell me repeatedly is that the message they get from courts on how to prevent malpractice suits is to perform more c-sections and to perform them early. Surgical birth becomes the answer to preventing liability threats, even though there is little evidence that c-sections prevent most bad outcomes.

I also commonly heard about the role of professional workshops and conferences. As I mentioned just a few pages ago, these workshops and conferences teach maternity providers the importance of documentation in preventing liability threats. However, the messages from these workshops and conferences go beyond documentation that protocols were diligently followed. Physicians talk about how these types of conferences affect how they assess risk in labor. Physician Philip Burgin speaks about a workshop he attended in which a prominent malpractice insurance plaintiffs' attorney lectured: "One of the plaintiffs' lawyers said something I [will] never [forget]: 'OK, if you're thinking about a c-section, you should be doing a c-section.'" Similarly, physician Lois Timberlake tells me of a lecture she attended at a professional conference: "There was one lecture I heard at a New England ob-gyn society meeting. . . . He started out as an obstetrician, and then he got his law degree, and he was very much, 'When in doubt, section . . . don't even think twice about it.'" In other words, attorneys spread fear of bad outcomes *and* c-section as an answer to this fear.

Litigating attorneys also spread fear of liability by seeking potential clients through advertising on local radio and television stations. Physicians commonly spoke about litigation attorneys' television commercials that target them for malpractice lawsuits. Physician Rosemary Steel tells me, "I'm sure you've seen those commercials with the lawyers saying, 'Is your child not as smart as you think [she] should be? Maybe it was a birth injury. Why don't you give us a call?' I mean, those kinds of commercials, of course, drive me crazy because they're picking on things that don't even exist sometimes." These types of media presentations are perceived as threatening to maternity providers.

Once this definition of c-sections as relief to liability threats takes hold, the definition spreads among providers, even those who have not been sued. I heard this sentiment countless times in my interviews; it seems to be an unwavering belief among all types of maternity providers—nurses, midwives, and physicians—here expressed by physician Maggie Rust: "There is a whole perception that if you have a bad outcome but you've done a c-section that you're not as much at risk being the physician as you are if you had a bad outcome and you had a vaginal delivery."

Are C-Sections Just More Convenient for Obstetricians?

It is important here to digress for just a moment to examine the idea that physicians perform c-sections out of convenience, something that is heard in everyday conversation. I argue that convenience should be understood within the organizational constraints physicians face. For example, physicians would likely rather do c-sections outside of office hours rather than attend vaginal births during office hours because they need to see patients to earn money to pay skyrocketing malpractice premiums. Most health insurance companies pay a global fee for birth. That means that health insurance companies pay the physician a single rate, usually between $2,500 and $3,500, for all prenatal visits and the birth. Physicians are not compensated for attending a long labor, and if a physician interrupts office hours to attend a birth, he or she will potentially lose money by not seeing scheduled patients. Remember, as malpractice insurance premiums escalate, obstetricians must see more and more patients just to cover that increased rate. Protecting office hours becomes a necessity. Further, although providers performing c-sections in the evening may seem to smack of convenience, it is also the case that evening c-sections allow providers not to miss any office hours and to sleep at night. Getting a good night's sleep is in the interest of providers who, because of increasing malpractice insurance rates, feel a pressure to see patients as many days in the week as possible. Many maternity providers told me they often have a full slate of patients, even if they were on the call the night before. Obstetricians also expressed concern about the safety of c-sections during the nighttime because everyone is likely to be more tired.

In other words, liability may underlie "convenience" because of the pressure to earn money to pay malpractice insurance premiums. It may be that some physicians are performing c-sections to go play golf or to go to dinner, but with most physicians operating in group practices, this is not as much of a concern as it used to be with solo practices. In short, organizational constrains are a better explanation of practices that seem to be convenient for physicians.

Conclusion

"My goal is that everybody goes home healthy and happy, and I don't get sued. . . . That's my goal. And maybe I get paid. . . . Everybody's happy. . . . For me that's a perfect case," Physician Philip Burgin tells me toward the end of the interview. Maternity providers have learned from courts, conferences, professional organizations, hospitals, insurers, and the media that the way to prevent liability threats is to perform c-sections. Organizational structures define c-sections as an answer to the liability threats faced by maternity providers. The rule of anticipated reaction is in play. Maternity providers try to avoid negative consequences by jumping quickly to c-sections. This is a way that organizations control behavior, even though it may not be apparent that organizations are behind individuals' decisions. As physician Jack Bianco tells me:

> So why not? . . . We're not stupid. You kick us long enough, we respond. Do we believe in it? No. Do I believe we're doing far too many c-sections? Absolutely. But every once in a while, you'll try to let someone labor longer, even if it's unpredictable because nature's unpredictable, shoulder events, something will happen, and we'll get blamed for it. So until society decides it doesn't want to put up with this anymore, we're going to continue to move in this direction because that's what society has asked us to do.

Organizations have responded to uncertain legal, political, and economic environments, and one response that has coalesced among organizations has been to define c-sections as the gold standard for a "safe" birth.

Still, women do not commonly perceive that their births are being held in the hands of providers who feel backed into a corner. They trust their doctors and believe that if they recommend a c-section, it must be necessary. The Listening to Mothers II Survey found that, while 62 percent of women believe that the current malpractice system causes providers to take better care of their patients, well less than half believe that providers would perform an unnecessary c-section to avoid being sued.[41] Trust in providers was a common sentiment, here expressed in the words of Dianne, a thirty-four-year-old woman who delivered her second child by c-section after two hours of pushing failed to result in a vaginal birth: "I mean I'm happy. The baby is safe, and I'm OK. I was avoiding a c-section. . . . I had to go through all possible ways of having a vaginal delivery, but I still couldn't get a vaginal delivery. Yeah, so it was a little disappointing, but at the end all that matters is a healthy baby and healthy me, of course. Right?" What would women like Dianne think if they knew how preoccupied their providers are with being blamed for a bad outcome? Would they so easily discount their desire for a vaginal birth?

PART II

Control Systems Embedded in Hospitals

2

The Tyranny of the Rules

I had a patient once who . . . tried to refuse fetal monitoring, and the nurse became irate and . . . she refused. She basically said . . . "I can't do that. I won't do that for you. This is my license. . . . If something bad happens here, it's my license."

—Midwife Rita Morey

Midwife Morey's tale gives us a glimpse into how women experience birth in hospitals. Their choices are determined by protocols, or rules for care of patients, put in place by hospital administrators, voted on by nurses and physicians, but based on organizational recommendations, typically ACOG and risk management departments of hospitals. Protocols guide the standard of care, which is considered the minimum care a provider is expected to give. Maternity providers feel they must strictly follow protocols to protect themselves from a lawsuit in the case of a bad outcome. In short, a breech of protocols defines medical error, and faithfully following protocols reduces liability risk to maternity providers and hospitals.

Empirical research supports the idea that following protocols protects one from liability in the case of a bad outcome. For example, Ransom and colleagues in a 2003 article published in *Obstetrics and Gynecology* found that 80 percent of delivery-related malpractice claims involved the departure from defined "pathways" of care, and when compared to cases in which a claim was not filed, noncompliance with a defined clinic pathway led to nearly a sixfold increase in the odds that a malpractice claim would be filed.[1]

Much work in organizational theory focuses on the human factor in organizations or the fact that humans are reflective and, thus, difficult to control in an organizational setting.[2] In particular, humans bring their own set of values and ideas into organizations, and these values and ideas may not align with organizational goals. As a consequence, organizations constantly struggle to secure the cooperation of organizational actors (e.g., employees, clients, customers) in working toward organizational goals. Although many organizational theories discuss this tension, probably the best elaborated discussion of how organizations deal with the human factor in organizations is the decision-making theory of Herbert Simon, Richard Cyert, and James March.[3] These theorists suggest that for individuals to make decisions in line with organizational goals and for organizational rationality to emerge, particularly under conditions of environmental uncertainty, organizational mechanisms are used to make congruent the decisions of the organizational actor with the organization's interests.[4] One of these mechanisms is the development of routines implemented around common decisions such that individuals do not have to decide the actions to take upon each new decision-making opportunity.[5] Rather, decisions are constrained in such a way to bring into line the actions and decisions of organizational actors with the goals of the organization.

There are many common examples of how this happens. In the case of the Washington DC school cheating scandal I discussed in the introduction, the teachers and principals were given organizational incentives (bonuses) to increase test scores. When I discussed decision-making theory in one of my classes a few years ago, one of my students, who was also a Starbucks employee, brought in an employee manual that instructed employees how to make the company's signature drinks, how to serve them, and what to say to customers. There was no doubt about exactly how much of each ingredient to put in the blender, in what order, and how to present the drink to the customer. Further, as George Ritzer suggests in his infamous book *The McDonaldization of Society*, the behavior of employees in a range of places, from restaurants to insurance companies to daycare centers, are constrained within very tight limits.[6]

This type of control over decisions also happens in hospitals. Hospital administrators are concerned about liability, and they put protocols in place that define expected behavior in such a way that the actions and decisions of individuals within hospitals are constrained to make malpractice claims less likely. This is done by hospital administrators' and committees' carefully defining appropriate actions in almost every aspect of monitoring, treating, and caring for women during labor and birth. If these rules are closely followed, maternity providers and hospital administrators believe they will not be blamed in the case of a bad birth outcome. I will demonstrate in this chapter that because all decisions about birth involve some risk and an opportunity for the maternity provider to make the "wrong" decision and to be held responsible for it, choices become increasingly narrowed so that fewer and fewer "bad decisions" can be made. This is accomplished by hospitals' setting protocols. Protocols can be seen as control systems put in place by organizations to deal with liability threats in uncertain economic, political, and legal environments.

Maternity providers' strictly following protocols would not be concerning—perhaps it would even be comforting—if protocols were shown to make labor and birth safer or to improve outcomes. However, only one-third of ACOG recommendations are based on "good and consistent" scientific evidence.[7] Further, researchers have concluded that a small cadre of physicians who regularly serve as expert witnesses for plaintiffs in bad-birth-outcome cases often influence the standard of care because hospital administrators closely watch the results of lawsuits and often change protocols based on the outcomes of court cases.[8] This is important to understand also because the physicians testifying in court tend to be older male physicians who do not participate much in clinical care and have few academic publications to their name.[9] What this means is that a few physicians, whose expertise is not based on recent clinical or research experience, influence the defined standard of care. This finding indicates the extent to which the legal system sets the rules of the game and takes decision making away from maternity providers and women.

I also show in this chapter how these control systems differently affect organizational actors depending on their positions. So, whereas I argued in chapter 1 that maternity providers think about the liability in much the same way—they are fearful—you will see that conflict still emerges among nurses, midwives, and physicians. Each group of individuals has different constraints on their behavior and actions because of their organizational locations. The important thing to notice is that the conflicts often are quite vehement and, in the end, the winning solution tends to move women closer and closer to a c-section.

The Patient Safety Movement

To understand the link between strictly following protocols and the rise in the c-section rate, it is important to understand the influence of the patient safety movement on hospital protocols. This movement stems from attention paid to a 1999 Institute of Medicine (IOM) report on the amount of human error present in the U.S. medical system, suggesting that between forty-four thousand and ninety-eight thousand deaths each year are attributable to preventable medical errors.[10] The report was a call to arms to revamp safety in medical care, and one of the focuses has become preventing adverse obstetric events. The approach that has developed as applied to obstetrics and advocated by obstetricians within the patient safety movement, notably Doctor Stephen Clark, involves: (1) standardization of process and protocol to "clearly define one way in which the standard of care may be met"; (2) standardization of language; (3) peer review and collaboration; and (4) the cesarean section rate not being defined as an outcome measure of quality.[11] Bill Barth, chair of the ACOG Practice Committee, describes the movement this way:

> I guess the best is an analogy to the airline industry. For years, the airline industry has had formal programs in safety that include specific activities like standardized emergency checklists, simulation training in the conduct of emergencies, uniform policies for the conduct of normal flight operations, extensive review of adverse outcomes. . . . Medicine at large . . . [has] turned towards this type of a process

There is no doubt that medical errors occur across every medical care specialty, but as I have argued earlier in the book, obstetrics is a special case. Medical errors may be committed in obstetrics, but the majority of negative birth outcomes are due to unpreventable events, such as shoulder dystocia, and unpreventable conditions, such as cerebral palsy. Thus it should not come as a surprise that the obstetric patient safety literature, in which obstetricians are the main authors, focuses more on preventing malpractice claims than on making birth safer, and the defined way of preventing malpractice claims in the minds of providers is to jump more quickly to a c-section.[12] In other words, the obstetricians who fear being sued are in charge of the obstetrical patient safety movement. This is rather akin to the fox guarding the chicken house. Perhaps this is why when safety protocols were implemented at Yale Hospital the c-section rate went up.[13]

The irony here is that in maternity care one of the main reasons maternal deaths are on the rise is that more c-sections are being performed.[14] Any practice that plays a part in elevating the national c-section rate over 15 percent contributes to maternal death. The patient safety movement has contributed to the increasing c-section epidemic, yet this epidemic stands in stark contrast to "safety" in birth. Thus I cannot help but be somewhat skeptical of this movement in obstetrics, although, understandably, it is difficult to argue against "patient safety." I will show how the patient safety movement as it has played out in obstetrical care can be seen as an attempt by ACOG, hospital administrators, and maternity providers to deal with uncertain legal, political, and economic environments and liability threats. Instead of making birth safer, it has led to more maternal deaths by driving up the c-section rate. The emphasis of the patient safety movement may apply better to other units of the hospital, but the safest thing in labor and birth is usually less, not more, intervention and individualized care, not standardization. In short, this movement in obstetrics is *not* first and foremost about patient safety in obstetrics.

Standardization

Let me start with the first pillar of the movement: the standardization of process and protocol so that there becomes one "best" way of delivering care.[15] Although the patient safety movement did not create standard protocols in modern-day labor and birth, the movement has exacerbated the *importance* of standardization.[16] Standardization of medical care is noted by medical scholars to have first been pushed forward for managerial purposes that are consistent with federal and legalistic control of medicine.[17] Much of the reason for increased standardization since 1983 in all medical procedures is due to Congress' mandating in 1982 that Medicare implement a prospective payment system. Such a system required that Medicare reimburse hospitals a flat fee for services based on diagnosis-related groups (DRGs). The change was championed as a way to rein in health care costs by incentivizing hospitals to be more efficient. But, as Rosemary Stevens, a noted historian of medicine, wrote in her book *In Sickness and in Wealth: American Hospitals in the Twentieth Century*, the change also served to standardize hospital work and protocols, in a way reminiscent of scientific management or Taylorism.[18]

Stevens also argues that standardization instills a sense of distrust between medical providers and patients because it promotes the idea that there is only one way of doing things, and straying from that one way may be perceived by patients as a medical error even when the course of action is deemed best by the provider based on his or her experience, knowledge, and training.[19] Standardization simplifies decisions, and, in doing so, does not allow medical providers to take into account complex factors that may be difficult to quantify, such as a patient's tolerance for pain and general preferences.[20] As midwife Crystal Hereford tells me, "Patients aren't all the same, and women aren't all the same, and labors aren't all the same."

Standardization is a well-established principle in labor and delivery, yet few of the protocols are based on good scientific evidence. Rather, I argue that standardization meets organizational imperatives of hospitals to reduce liability threats. An indication that standardized protocols are tied to reducing liability threats is the fact that hospitals may change protocols very quickly in response to lawsuits or a hospital's or maternity provider's bad experience with a negative birth outcome.[21] Physicians talk in general about this trend of integrating past bad outcomes into protocols. For example, physician Jack Bianco tells me, "The standard of care changed because we do things to make big jury decision lawsuits less feasible, and we do things to better document our ability to defend what we do. That's what the standard of care has changed to reflect." Physician Jacob Chism echoes this sentiment: "Protocols specify the frequency of documentation and what needs to be documented. . . . Some of it is good care, but some of it is malpractice and defensibility and that sort of thing."

I was told tales of specific instances of changes to protocols as a reaction to a bad outcome or a lawsuit. Most changes make vaginal birth more difficult to attain and c-section more likely. What follows are two telling examples of how this occurs:

> We had a low-risk patient walking the halls. Early, early, early stages of labor. Probably could have gone home, but for whatever [reason] . . . maybe her pain level, whatever, they opted to keep her. She walks the halls, gets back into bed. There is no heartbeat for absolutely no explainable reason. . . . It's one more reason to keep everybody on [the electronic fetal monitor] all the time. (Nurse Amanda Barnett)

> I was a labor and delivery nurse before I went to midwifery school. And the year before I came there, [Community] Hospital had one of the biggest lawsuits . . . in the history of the state of Connecticut. . . . Basically, it was a twenty-cent piece of plastic . . . tubing that [wasn't] connected, and the baby didn't get oxygen, and so the baby had CP [cerebral palsy], and it truly was negligent. . . . I came on as a labor and delivery nurse a year or two later, [and]. . . . they had stricter rules about . . . when the doctor

had to show up, how long a person had to be on the fetal monitor, and it was because they had this really horrible experience and this big lawsuit that made the front page of all the state newspapers. I am quite sure, after that happened and they made all these really strict rules for laboring women, . . . their c-section rate went up. . . . The interesting thing is . . . that they do this knee-jerk response . . . not really based in science. It's just this overreaction that something happened. . . . They made all these crazy, crazy rules that had nothing to do with the fact that there was this bad outcome. . . . And a lot of the changes . . . [made] it hard for women to have [a] normal [vaginal] delivery. (Midwife Crystal Hereford)

In other words, protocols may be changed in reaction to one bad outcome, hardly an evidence-based decision-making process, although such a reaction may seem rational to hospital administrators who are trying to reduce liability threats. It is important to note from both examples that ACOG guidelines set the standards that are followed, but the standards may become stricter than ACOG recommendations when hospitals react to bad outcomes. Often, the changes make it more difficult for women to have vaginal births.

A specific example of a protocol change that makes c-section more likely but that is not based on sound evidence of improved outcomes is routine c-section for babies presenting in a breech position. "Nobody knows how to do vaginal breech deliveries anymore" physician Molly Nichols laments to me on a sunny summer afternoon in my office. Doctor Nichols is clearly frustrated by the current state of birth and tells me this in an exasperated voice. She is right that few breech babies are delivered vaginally. Nearly 90 percent of babies in breech position were delivered by c-section in 2010.[22] In my data, two women had babies presenting in a breech position, and both had scheduled c-sections.

Physician James Montenegro tells me of a surprise vaginal breech delivery he had recently attended:

I did one personally . . . a couple months ago. I happened to be the in-house doc. There was no other doc around. A clinic patient rolled in. . . . She was a multip [she had given birth at least once before]. She comes in fully dilated with the butt on the perineum and to protect myself, I call my chairman . . . [and say], "I have no problem with this. It's a piece of cake. I just need you to say it's OK for me to do," because I couldn't get this kid out faster with a c-section. I could take her back for a c-section, but she would deliver before we got her back there. So, [I said to my chairman], "I just need your blessing that you'll support me on this." And he was so nervous . . . I said, "I don't need you here." He said, "I'll be there in five minutes." . . . I'm fifty-one years old; my chairman is forty-seven, forty-eight, and he's bouncing off the walls behind me. And I say, "Will you settle down? . . . And everyone applauded because they hadn't seen [a vaginal breech delivery] in so many years.

Even though Doctor Montenegro is comfortable with delivering a breech vaginally—he has the experience and skills necessary—notice his concern with having his chairman's approval so that he will be protected in the case of a bad outcome.

Physicians told me that the disappearance of vaginal breech deliveries is a direct attempt by hospital administrators and maternity providers to prevent liability. For example, physician Lawrence Rascon says:

[The shift to delivering breech babies by c-section] was done [all] because of liability concerns. . . . That's the only reason. . . . I mean, 95 percent of breeches could be delivered safely vaginally. But think about that. If 5 percent can't [and] if you're doing 100 breeches at a hospital in five years say . . . you're talking about five major lawsuits. So you've got to do a lot of sections to protect those few babies.

The decline in vaginal breech births did not come out of nowhere. A specific study—the Term Breech Trial, authored by Mary E. Hannah and colleagues and published in 2000—is linked to the drastic decline in this practice. This study included 26 countries, 121 hospitals, and 2,183 women who had babies in a breech position at term and were randomly assigned to have either a vaginal breech delivery or a c-section.[23] The study found that breech babies born vaginally fared worse at two months of age than did breech babies born by c-section. This study nearly shut down vaginal breech births worldwide.[24] Yet the tide turned too quickly because the study has been heavily criticized for its methodology and its findings called into question.[25] For example, researchers have demonstrated that the neonatal deaths that occurred in the study population were not related to mode of delivery.[26] Further, a follow-up study by the original authors published in 2004 shows that the difference in outcome detected between babies born vaginally and babies born by c-section at two months of age was not present when children were examined at two years of age—the children fared the same.[27] In short, the standard of care changed based on highly criticized research, and its findings were integrated into ACOG and *Cochrane Review* guidelines.[28]

Maternity providers commonly mentioned this study to me as a constraining factor to their support of vaginal breech delivery. Physician Arthur Berkowitz describes the effect of the Term Breech Trial: "A common sentiment I think that you'll hear is, 'Well I'm trained in doing [a vaginal breech delivery], and I'm comfortable in doing it, but there are occasionally going to be bad outcomes, and now that the Hannah [Term Breech] Trial has been published, [if] I do it and there's a bad outcome, I'm toast.'" This is the effect, even though delivering a baby presenting in a breech position by c-section increases the risk to the mother compared to planned vaginal delivery and the findings from the Term Breech Trial have been largely discredited.[29]

Some critical researchers suggest that even though the Term Breech Trial had obvious errors, ACOG did not question those errors because the findings were exactly what the obstetrical community was hoping for. According to Marek Glezerman in a paper he wrote criticizing the Term Breech Trial:

> The recommendations of the [Term Breech Trial] were not only awaited anxiously by obstetricians of mainly Western countries but also almost gratefully accepted. It is much easier to plan an abdominal delivery than a vaginal delivery, and it requires less expertise to do so. Moreover, in the current medico–legal environment, in which litigation for a performed cesarean section is a rare event but vaginal delivery carries increased risks for litigation, obstetricians easily can be convinced not to take this risk. Consequently, the conclusions of the [Term Breech Trial] are perceived today by many obstetricians as a badly needed set of arguments for [primary cesarean section], which they would have preferred anyway.[30]

It seems, then, that liability concerns may be at the root of the widespread acceptance of this study and its implications.

It is not only vaginal breech delivery of individual babies that has gone by the wayside because of liability concerns. The hesitance to perform vaginal breech deliveries is extended to vaginal twin deliveries, especially because in many cases one of the twins is in a breech position. This is concerning because there is no evidence that delivering a twin that is not presenting head down by c-section rather than vaginally improves the baby's outcome.[31] Physician Arthur Berkowitz suggests that the threshold for c-section has crept lower and that vaginal breech twin birth is a good example of how that happens:

> Basically what [the Term Breech Trial] did was stop people in North America and probably worldwide actually from performing purposeful vaginal breech deliveries. And that study got a lot of press and really heavily swayed practice. . . . The practice has changed so permanently in that regard I don't think anyone will ever go back. . . . What happened there was I think this sort of, actually I'm trying to think of a word to call it—let's call it creep of the threshold. . . . If you know that the Term Breech Trial is out there and that vaginal breech is no longer advised, if you have a second twin that's breech or transverse and might end up breech, you're less likely to be as aggressive with twins. So I think that the Term Breech Trial negatively began to impact practitioners willing to perform twin deliveries vaginally, and I know private hospitals where just all twins are sectioned because of that. Yet it's not a good application of the science because that's not what the Term Breech Trial addressed.

Further, the vicious cycle of providers not wanting to take the risk of a vaginal twin delivery because of liability concerns and the small risk of a negative outcome means that obstetrical residents are unlikely to receive training on how to perform them. This undoubtedly increases the c-section rate because the rate of twins has soared in the United States over the past thirty years by 77 percent, from 18.9 per 1,000 live births in 1980 to 33 per 1,000 live births in 2010.[32] In our data, two women had twin pregnancies. Both women had c-sections—one had a scheduled c-section and one attempted a vaginal birth but eventually had a c-section. Doctor Berkowitz goes on to talk about the problem to which lack of training leads:

> On the practitioner side, if we're not doing planned vaginal breech deliveries anymore, very few people are getting trained in them. What it . . . come[s] down to [is] being able to sit across from a patient [who] you care about and have bonded with and tell them, "I'll be there for you to deliver your second twin as a breech." [This] is harder to do if you haven't done breech deliveries. So, those kind of maneuvers, forceps, and breech deliveries, those skills are not being taught at the same rate and volume that they were previously, and so more recent practitioners are not as comfortable with those.

Physician Christopher Froehlich concurs with Doctor Berkowitz's assessment of the lack of training and extends it to encompass vaginal birth of any breech baby—singleton or twins—when he tells me, "If you ask most young obstetricians, 'Do you feel more comfortable doing a breech birth vaginally or a c-section?' I would say 95 percent of them would say, 'Oh, no question, c-section.'" This lack of training is important because even if the liability threat is addressed, few providers will be trained in how to perform vaginal breech and twin deliveries, condemning women to a c-section even if the nonsurgical options are redefined as "safe." Physician Lawrence Rascon says:

> There [are] almost no obstetricians now [who] are trained . . . to deliver breech babies [vaginally]. . . . When I was a resident, we did breech delivery vaginally. . . . But . . . my partners [who] are younger, even five or seven years younger than me, . . . they're not comfortable doing the procedure. Even if legally it [were] safer, they wouldn't be able to do the procedure because of that.

In other words, without concerted effort vaginal breech delivery may never come back as a practice.

Beyond vaginal delivery of breech babies is the possibility of changing the position of a breech baby in utero to a head-down or cephalic presentation through a procedure called external cephalic version or ECV for short. In this procedure, while the fetal heartbeat pattern is carefully monitored, ultrasound technology is used to help maternity providers manually push and pull the fetus into a head-down presentation. The *Cochrane Review* of this procedure shows its success in turning babies head down and facilitating a vaginal birth and finds that negative effects of the procedure happen so rarely that they are hard to capture in empirical research.[33] Yet ECV is a waning practice. Many providers told me that ECV simply creates more risk than hospital administrators and maternity providers will tolerate. Midwife Pam Grays used the decline of this procedure to illustrate to me an example of how fear guides protocol changes:

> There was a case a few years ago here where one of our doctors performed a version, and it was successful, and it went really well, and the protocol at the time was that you monitor the baby for, I think it's either two or four hours following the procedure, just to make sure that the baby has tolerated the procedure well. And then the patient was sent home, and I think

she ended up coming back later that day or the next day, and her baby had died, sadly. . . . It certainly wasn't directly a cause from the version itself, because everything had checked out. . . . Since then, the protocol at this hospital . . . has changed that now if a patient has a successful version, they have to be immediately induced, and if the version is unsuccessful, then they immediately go for a c-section. So, that one case, which may or may not really hold merit, has really changed completely, in this hospital, the procedure for versions and also it ended up affecting significantly the success rates of doing a version, because you can't do it too soon, because if you are going to induce the patient afterwards, you can't induce somebody who is preterm. But if you wait too long, then the version is going to have very little success [because the baby will be too big to rotate].

Physician Dale Samaniego also brought up ECV and how it is related to risk that a provider may fear:

It's a lot of liability, it's a lot of time, and it can be risky. Sometimes you try and vert [change the baby to a vertex or head-down presentation] somebody, and you vert them, and then they monitor them for a little bit, and you send them home, and then they come back and let's say they have a baby, it passes away because of a cord problem. . . . I don't think you're going to see a lot of versions in private practice because it's just not worth it.

I question whether women would view the risk of ECV in the same way. The most recent scientific review on this procedure concludes as follows: "The review of seven studies, 1,245 women, found that if the baby is not head down after about 36 weeks of pregnancy, ECV reduces the chance that the baby will present as breech at the time of birth, and reduces the chance of caesarean birth."[34]

The bottom line is that women are not typically presented a choice in these situations but are told that they need to have a c-section. Standardization of protocols direct maternity providers' decisions and actions, but the protocols may be so constricting that maternity providers are not allowed to facilitate vaginal birth. In other words, in modern-day maternity care, standardization often prevents providers from doing things that are intended to help women deliver vaginally. This is especially concerning given that few protocols are based on sound scientific evidence of improved fetal or maternal outcomes and are more closely tied to legal decisions and averting liability risk.

Standardization of Language

A second pillar of the patient safety movement is standardization of language. The place where this is most evident in modern maternity care is in how one interprets electronic fetal monitoring strips. The hot topic in CTG research is not how to prevent its overuse or how to develop other tests to assess fetal well-being, which clearly would be the strategy most beneficial to women, families, and the economic vitality of the health care system, but rather on how to "correctly" interpret the strips.[35] The National Institute of Child Health and Human Development (NICHD) sponsored a Research Planning Workshop in 2008 that addressed the standardization of language in the interpretation of CTG results.[36] The classification system developed includes three categories of CTG tracings: Category I (Normal), Category II (Intermediate), and Category III (Abnormal).[37] Category I tracings are considered reassuring, while Category III tracings are non-reassuring and indicative of the need for immediate delivery. The problem is that most tracings fall into Category II, where the discretion of maternity providers is highest.[38] In fact, experts in CTG suggest that to understand how to interpret these categories, clinicians should learn how to identify Category I and Category III tracings, because all the other tracings are, by default, Category II tracings.[39] The new classification system that has developed out of the patient safety movement has created more ambiguity about the tracings and left the majority of readings difficult to interpret, what Yale obstetrics professors Christian Pettker and Charles Lockwood refer to as "wiggle room."[40]

There is no doubt that effective communication is important in providing appropriate medical care to patients. However, it seems odd for so much focus to be placed on standardizing the language used for an ineffective technology. This peculiarity is likely due to the tie of the standardization of language to an attempt to decrease liability threat. Physician Jeffrey Starling's words support the link to reducing liability:

I think it has helped a lot to at least have everybody interpret things in the same way and, therefore, not either over- or under-interpret tracings, and it was part of our patient safety program, and it had a lot of wonderful beneficial facts for that and many less adverse outcomes. We've had no obstetrical malpractice claims in three years, et cetera, et cetera. And then our section rate has gone from 22 percent when I got here in 2002 to about 34 percent [in 2010].

Physician Starling's linking together the standardization of protocols to decreasing malpractice claims is a common association made by maternity providers. But doing so strikes me as a logical fallacy. I highlight this logical fallacy, not to criticize physician Starling, who is a thoughtful physician quite concerned about the increasing c-section rate, but rather to point out the importance of thinking critically about the effect of the patient safety movement on c-sections. As social scientists are fond of saying, correlation is not necessarily causation. In other words, two trends—like, for example, the number of storks in a country and that country's birth rate— may be correlated.[41] Yet we know that storks don't really bring babies. The two trends are correlated, but one is not causing the other. Similarly, the link between the standardization of protocols and a lack of obstetrical malpractice claims may not be causally related. Bad outcomes are rare, and it may be months or years between bad outcomes and malpractice lawsuits (which are often filed years after a bad outcome). Yet, if the standardization of protocols (and an increase in the c-section rate) occurs during a period of good outcomes and no malpractice lawsuits, the two trends may become causally linked in the minds of providers who are hoping to prevent bad outcomes *and* malpractice law suits. However, there is no proof that the standardized protocols *cause* the lack of bad outcomes or lawsuits.

Dr. Andrew Robinette echoes the focus of liability in the shift in nomenclature, suggesting that physicians take classes on nomenclature as a defensive move:

> One of our defenses . . . is we've . . . made every one of our . . . 160 physicians and midwives and nurse–practitioners take a course on standard nomenclature in fetal monitoring. . . . We had a case where . . . a midwife or a nurse would talk to a physician on the telephone, and they weren't talking the same formalities. So everybody has to be on the same page. . . . I also want to say when any one of my physicians get sued, "Guess what? They just went through this standardized program. Here's our certificate. Here's what they had to do." You know, it's also medical/legal.

There is no doubt from a commonsense perspective that it is good for everyone to be on the same page and to understand one another. Yet the motivating factor pushing this standardization is not about improving patient care, but rather about how everyone's being up-to-date on nomenclature may prevent a lawsuit in the case of a bad outcome. It seems especially counterintuitive for the patient safety movement to focus on the standardization of language involving a clearly ineffective technology, further promulgating its use. Empirical research suggests that outcomes are just as good when women are monitored intermittently with a handheld Doppler unit and that the use of continuous CTG increases a woman's chance of having a c-section.[42]

Peer Review and Collaboration

A third mechanism of the patient safety movement is peer review and collaboration. Peer review is an established mechanism in which a committee of physicians evaluates a specific case to decide whether the physician followed the standard of care. Collaboration, on the other hand, refers to physicians, midwives, and nurses working together as a team to monitor women and babies. These sound like good ideas—who wouldn't want a team of professionals taking care of them and physicians regularly reviewed on how they care for patients? Yet what I heard about most in terms of collaboration is how it often keeps women from having a vaginal birth, and in terms of peer review is how reviews focus on bad outcomes that result from vaginal birth, reinforcing the view that c-sections are the preferred and "safer" (for the provider) mode of birth. I will focus in this section on collaboration because peer review is so closely tied to the topic I cover in the next section—not using c-section as a quality measure.

Let me explain how collaboration may lead to c-sections. Collaboration allows any person on the team to make a decision that a vaginal birth or an intervention's being used to help a woman attain a vaginal birth is not safe. Although collaboration is done in the name of safety, for maternity providers many times the ultimate motivation for implementing safety protocols is reducing liability threats. Physician Andrew Robinette explains how collaboration is inherently a defensive strategy:

> [The increased liability pressures are an] unsustainable situation. . . . And so we have introduced a culture of safety. . . . There's a collaborative model. . . . As I heard one plaintiff's attorney say, "It's easy to convince a jury that a good driver on a sunny day on a straight road in good weather went off into a ditch, but to convince them that two people did it on the same road on the same day—very tough." So, we always try to get a second opinion. . . . And then the second way is the c-section rate's gone up.

Physician Robinette explains that collaboration is a defensive move. Notice also how he suggests that the c-section rate increase is part and parcel of the culture of safety.

Physician Andrew Robinette also explains another way that collaboration can lead to c-sections. When physicians are not able to clearly articulate why they are comfortable continuing a vaginal birth attempt—when they cannot defend *inaction*—they move toward a c-section:

> We've also taught people to examine every action they do and say . . . "How will I be able to defend this action to others?" And a lot of times they'll say, "I just can't . . . I understand what I'm doing, but I can't explain it to anybody so I'm going to [do a c-]section."

Again, although it may seem counterintuitive, collaboration may not allow physicians to individualize care and to help women attain a vaginal delivery, although collaboration need not be structured this way. Collaboration could benefit women—for example, the collaboration of midwives and physicians to facilitate women having a vaginal birth, but that is not the current focus of collaboration in the patient safety movement.

The ways that collaboration can lead to c-sections plays out most commonly in three areas: the use of continuous electronic fetal monitoring, the use of Pitocin, and consultation with maternal–fetal medicine (MFM) specialists. I'll first discuss the use of electronic fetal monitors. Most hospitals have centralized monitoring, and every woman's labor is visible on monitors at a central location and sometimes in each labor and delivery room, making each woman's labor visible to all maternity providers. With the promotion of collaboration, other maternity providers—nurses, physicians, or midwives—may exert pressure to keep women on continuous CTG, thus increasing the chance of a c-section. The question may well be "Why is she off the monitor?" Physician Maggie Rust puts it this way: "It's not my choice to go in there and do something that isn't routine, that isn't acceptable in kind of the general form. The nurses are watching you; the residents are watching you; the staff is watching you."

Because of litigation concerns, this type of pressure can be quite extreme and stamp out the use of intermittent monitoring, as described by an experienced midwife, Crystal Hereford:

> We had this group of patients that didn't want to be on the fetal monitor, and it became this big brouhaha at [Community] Hospital. . . . It was

the same discussion that I've had a million times since I've been a midwife. . . . They would say, "But [Crystal], if you have three hours of a tracing, and that baby looked good, then if that patient sues you, you could say the baby looked good on the monitor. If all you have are intermittent auscultations, and then you have a bad outcome, then they're going to have all the ammunition in the world to sue you."

Midwife Hereford experienced pressure from her colleagues to keep women on a CTG monitor, and this is something that a number of maternity providers mentioned. Because of collaboration—of everyone's having the right to comment on anyone's patient—more women are monitored continuously because anyone can ask, "Why isn't she on the monitor?" The focus is on always being able to see how the baby is faring in labor, which continuous CTG allows. Intermittent monitoring with a Doppler unit is just as effective as CTG in monitoring the baby, but it does not allow for providers to see every beat of the baby's heart.[43] The problem, of course, is that continuous CTG increases a woman's chance of having a c-section.[44]

The use of Pitocin is also a hugely contentious issue that leads to conflict of doctors and midwives against nurses. Doctor Steven Clark, one of the biggest advocates in obstetrics of the patient safety movement, and colleagues argue in a 2009 article published in the *American Journal of Obstetrics and Gynecology* that the most common source of conflict between obstetricians and nurses is over the administration of Pitocin.[45] The use of Pitocin is tied to the heavy use of induction to begin a woman's labor and to the near-ubiquitous use of epidurals for labor pain relief. Pitocin and epidurals team up with the artificial time line many women face to achieve a vaginal birth. In short, many women may find that they "need" Pitocin augmentation to deliver vaginally. It has become an intervention used to help women achieve vaginal birth in the face of other interventions, a practice that is indicative of the medicalized environment women face when giving birth in the contemporary United States. Because patience and waiting for a vaginal birth is not always the plan, Pitocin seems to be a created necessity.

Patient safety connects to this because physicians may not be able to use Pitocin to facilitate a vaginal birth due to patient safety protocols.[46] Researchers find that women who have epidurals and receive a low dose of Pitocin to augment labor, like those doses advocated by the patient safety movement, have an increased risk of c-section.[47] That is, when women have epidurals, they may need a higher dose of Pitocin to deliver vaginally than is allowed under current widespread protocols.

Further, because of the patient safety movement, nurses are empowered to turn off Pitocin, not to increase Pitocin, or not to administer Pitocin, even when physicians order Pitocin to help a woman achieve a vaginal delivery.[48] It is not that nurses are inherently more supportive of the protocols, but they are responsible for enforcing the protocols and face hospitals' firing them or not supporting them in a malpractice claim if they do not follow the protocols. If a physician or midwife wants to have the Pitocin increased but a nurse will not do this, the physician or midwife can go to the charge nurse and plead the case. The charge nurse will make a decision supporting either the nurse, or the physician or midwife. If she decides against the physician or midwife, he or she may then go to the attending physician or the most senior physician on call, who has the final word on whether Pitocin will be increased. Physician Jack Bianco tells me of his frustration with the current state of the use of Pitocin:

> Now there's this thing in medicine where anyone can stop the plane. So even the newest, youngest, most inexperienced nurse can stop Pitocin, even if I can justify on paper why it's safe to give, all she has to say is, "I'm uncomfortable giving it, and I can't give it." And the hospital is so scared that eventually when deposed, that nurse will say, "I was concerned about giving the Pit. The doctor made me do it," even if it's documented scientifically that it was safe to give.

Physician Bianco believes that collaboration increases the c-section rate because fear can drive decisions and, thus, he cannot use his expertise to facilitate a vaginal birth. I heard this theme often in the interviews, here from midwife Dorothy Lemert:

> Pitocin is a big one. . . . I have been in situations where we can't get the patient['s contractions] adequate because the nurse isn't doing her job [isn't increasing Pitocin often enough]. . . . You are not doing the patient any favors. You are prolonging the time it takes for a patient to go into labor.

Nurses, predictably, see this issue differently. Because they are responsible for administering Pitocin, they follow protocol. They know if they don't, they will be held responsible for a bad outcome:

[We have] the strength to say to a doctor, "I am not pitting [giving Pitocin to] her because when I am sitting in the chair and the judge asks me why, I will have no reason." And that's what . . . we say a lot of times when one of the residents says, "Well how come you didn't pit her?" "Because I have no defense. When I am sitting in the chair, I have no defense." (Nurse Amanda Barnett)

INTERVIEWER: Is that a rare occurrence that nurses will say "I'm not turn-ing Pitocin up"?
NURSE MARGIE NAPOLITANO: It's not rare. . . . It happens often . . . espe-cially because nurses are more vocal than they ever used to be, that we will say, "Well, I don't feel comfortable doing that."

Physicians and midwives have a few general responses to being denied the use of Pitocin to facilitate vaginal birth. One response is to do other inter-ventions to facilitate vaginal births. Midwife Dorothy Lemert tells me:

[Doing intervention is] what I have been forced to do to prevent c-sec-tions. I don't want to have to go in there and break the water and put an [intrauterine pressure catheter] in to make sure that their contractions are adequate to make sure that the nurses will go up on the Pitocin, but I do it because I know then [that] I have some objective data that the nurses are willing to look at and consider to go up on that Pitocin so that I can get a vaginal delivery.[49]

Another response of physicians and midwives is to wait until a shift change to find a nurse who will increase Pitocin.

Waiting for a shift change, going up the chain of command, or using other interventions in order to use or to increase Pitocin all take effort and time, and on a daily basis, some providers simply will not or cannot exert the time and energy to do so. This might explain the most common re-sponse I heard to what physicians do when a nurse will not carry out an or-der to give a woman Pitocin or to increase the dose of Pitocin, a response that I, perhaps naively, found shocking the first time I heard it—physicians "give up" and perform c-sections they feel are unnecessary. This frustrates some physicians, like Jack Bianco:

I'm clearly not having fun anymore. I'm fifty-seven, and I never thought I would ever want to stop practice, but I'm looking to be able to stop practice right now because it's such bullshit. It's such bullshit. I mean, I could be sitting there, and [the] nurse says [she won't increase Pitocin], and I can go up the chain of command, quote unquote, to the "most experienced doctor in charge," and the doctor says, "My hands are tied, it's protocol, we can't do it." Then [I say], "I'll do a c-section. I can't do anything about it. I guess I'll do a c-section."

Some physicians, like Lois Timberlake, are more resigned than angry:

I helped with a c-section the other night where the physician . . . wanted to give [his patient] Pitocin augmentation. And the nurses essentially said, "We are not comfortable with this tracing. We will not give Pitocin." And now, if he had pressed the point, there is a series of steps. . . . They would have called the nursing supervisor, who would have called the department chair, and this and that. . . . [He] just said, "Oh, I'm not going to fight this. What do you want me to do? Just section her? OK. Fine."

Still others, like physician Philip Burgin, are not bothered by performing c-sections when Pitocin may have helped a woman achieve a vaginal delivery, but see it as on par for the environment in which they find themselves:

I'm not a cowboy. I don't go outside the protocols. I try to get the best results and the best deliveries within the guidelines that have been set up so I don't create too much trouble. Because, remember, . . . the point of pushing the Pitocin to the extreme is to try to get a vaginal delivery. That's not my goal. My goal is to get a good result. So whether we have a vaginal delivery that happens easily or a c-section because she didn't get far into labor doesn't matter to me that much; my goal is not a vaginal delivery.

The reaction of physicians to strict enforcement of protocols is different, likely due to a divergence in their underlying commitment to vaginal birth, but they see the same issue, that collaboration prevents them from helping women attain vaginal births and leads to more and more c-sections.

Another form of collaboration that leads to more interventions and c-sections is when physicians and midwives feel compelled to consult MFM specialists. Maternal–fetal medical specialists are obstetricians who go through an additional three years of training in the medical and surgical management of high-risk pregnancies. Many maternity providers tell me that MFM doctors are likely to see pregnancy as dangerous because of their training and their experience seeing mostly women who have pregnancies that have some defined risk. Yet the collaborative model of care sometimes compels obstetricians and midwives to consult with MFM specialists when women, for example, are overdue or have suspected low amniotic fluid levels. I heard numerous times in my interviews that referrals are used as a "CYA" (cover your ass) strategy—"I talked to someone else." They told me that it is very common for MFM specialists to suggest inductions to deliver babies even when the obstetricians feel it would be reasonable for women to continue their pregnancies:

> A lot of times our high-risk doctors, the MFM doctors, . . . basically say that they recommend that we do an induction for whatever reason. And then in that way, you're kind of [bound] to do it because you've asked a specialist to help you manage this case and . . . they've given their opinion that you should induce the person. . . . I don't always agree with them, but at the same time, they're the specialists that I counseled to help manage my patient. So, you kind of get [bound] into doing something sometimes. (Physician Rosemary Steel)

Midwife Jill Wayland recounts a conversation she had with an obstetrician about how MFM physicians had taken over much decision-making responsibility in labor and delivery:

> I remember once saying to one of the older obstetricians, . . . we had this conversation—something was going on, I don't remember what it was. And he was sort of disgusted, like, "Since when was that a criteria for doing this?" And we were going to have to do . . . some kind of [intervention], and he said, "We didn't used to have to do that." And I said to him, "Tell me, why is it that . . . our MFM consultants are making all the decisions? . . . You guys used to make these decisions yourself." And he said, "Yeah . . . but with the legal system, . . . if an MFM doctor says I should do something and I don't do it, I'm dead, you know? So you have to do it."

Midwife Jill Wayland was so frustrated with the situation that she told me she planned to advise her daughter-in-law, if she becomes pregnant, to give birth in a hospital without MFM doctors on staff. She was going to make it her own job to find the right hospital for her daughter-in-law. She felt very strongly about this.

In these ways, I see unintended consequences of collaboration—that collaboration leads to more c-sections because it is a mechanism that allows the spread of liability fear. This is particularly the case with the phenomenon of "groupthink," a process documented to affect decisions of groups. This happens when groups become cohesive and begin to ignore disconfirming opinions and alternative courses of action.[50] Fear of a bad outcome may take over and lead to a consensus that interventions, like induction or a c-section, are necessary. People in the group who question the decision and feel that a wait-and-see attitude is more appropriate may not voice that view because it goes against the consensus in the group. This is a particular concern when fear is foremost in the minds of maternity providers, and this does seem to be the case currently. I am not arguing that collaboration necessarily leads to these results and that collaboration is never in a patient's interest. Research shows that collaboration, particularly of midwives and physicians, can lead to better birth outcomes.[51] But in the current legal and economic environment, the collaboration promoted by the patient safety movement seems to set in place practices and interventions that may lead to more c-sections.

"Cesarean Section" Is Not a Quality Measure

Hospitals also want to reduce risk, and they communicate this imperative in a few ways, all of which are tied to the fourth pillar of the patient safety movement—the c-section rate not being used as a quality measure. For example, Steven Clark and colleagues in their 2009 article in the *American Journal of Obstetrics and Gynecology* address the concern that a low-dose Pitocin protocol may increase the c-section rate: "We believe the time is long past when cesarean delivery rate can be considered a primary outcome of any importance."[52] As I will show in the following discussion, this move away from the c-section rate as a quality measure is a clear change from the past. Here is how physician Tony Oday describes the change:

> Your threshold for doing a c-section now today I think is a lot less than it was back fifteen, twenty years ago . . . [when] there was a lot of pressure at the time to do vaginal deliveries. And now it's just the opposite, where there is really no pressure whatsoever to try to keep your c-section rate low. No one is using that as a quality issue anymore when back then, fifteen, twenty years ago, . . . there were a lot of insurance companies,

hospitals, . . . saying well this a measure of quality of a physician—what his c-section rate is. So everyone wanted to try to get their c-section rate under 20 percent, and that pressure is not there anymore.

It is clear from physician Oday's statement that *not* using c-section rates as a measurement of quality leads to more c-sections.

The communication of organizational imperatives is accomplished in a number of ways, all of which notably leave out the c-section rate as a quality measure. For example, in grand rounds—a kind of lecture that is meant to educate medical students, in which physicians present information on particular patients, their treatments, and their outcomes—the imperative to prevent legal risk, not to prevent c-sections, is clearly communicated. Midwife Rosalie Batten gives me a specific example of grand rounds that communicates organizational priorities of hospitals to physicians and medical students:

We've had these discussions [at] . . . the grand rounds by a resident who talked about how many c-sections it would take to save one case of cerebral palsy, and it was a lot of c-sections, so you kind of walk away from that thinking, "Well, it really is ridiculous for us to be doing all these c-sections." But then she came back with, "But that one case of cerebral palsy is going to cost you, even if you settle out of court, a million dollars."

This clear communication of organizational imperatives lowers the threshold for performing c-sections.

Another way that hospitals indicate priorities to care providers is through hospital peer review. I was told that peer reviews almost always focus on bad outcomes. The definition of "bad outcome" is essential. I was told that it is rare for *maternal* injury to be reviewed as a bad outcome. The focus tends to be on injury to a *baby*. Further, because many of the consequences of c-sections to women are *future* consequences—reproductive consequences, bowel obstructions, and persistent pain—the negative outcomes of c-sections are missed. Thus, although women withstand the worst of the health costs of c-sections, these injuries often go unnoticed when *unnecessary* c-sections are not reviewed.[53] As Midwife Linville tells me, "If you have a bad outcome or low Apgars, or something, somebody's going to say, 'Why didn't you do a c-section?' But nobody ever looks at the other side of it when there's a uterine infection or bladder injury: 'Well, why was a c-section done in the first place?'"[54] This is in part a result of the patient safety movement's backing away from defining the c-section rate as a quality measure. The focus is on adverse obstetrical outcomes, typically for the baby, not on why a c-section was performed.

It is important that reviews have gone by the wayside because peer review of unnecessary c-sections sends a strong message to providers that it not acceptable to perform c-sections if a vaginal birth is possible. Physician Jeffrey Starling tells me of the deterrent effect of such reviews: "I've actually met with physicians and asked them about their . . . variation in their cesarean delivery rates and why are you always done by eleven at night? . . . They defend each case—the date was wrong, the analysis was wrong. And then when you present it to them, magically their section rate drops over the next year."

My concern is not only that c-sections aren't reviewed; I also am concerned that c-sections are being promoted in peer reviews as a way to prevent legal risk. Physician Jeffrey Starling goes on to describe this as a change: "The hospital then . . . reviews all these cases. They're going to . . . have to talk to a committee about why they *didn't* do a c-section. Of course, ten years ago they might have had to present why they *did* a section. It's going to change your attitude." Physician Lois Timberlake sees the same type of change that has happened, to the point that she wonders whether all *vaginal births* will soon be reviewed:

[Peer reviews are now] much more focused on bad outcomes. . . . I can still remember certain doctors getting up there and very pompously saying, "I don't think she was in active labor at this point even though she had been in labor for eighteen hours. I don't think she had gotten to active labor. I think you did a latent phase c-section." They would actually get very critical . . . and you would, when you're doing [a c-section] think, "Oh jeez, am I going to have to get up and at the next department meeting and explain this one away?" . . . [Now] everyone sits around there saying, "We should be reviewing the vaginal deliveries" . . . and "Why did you let this happen?" sort of jokingly but they're essentially saying, "We should have been looking, and why couldn't you have found a reason to do a c-section?"

This view may sound extreme, but numerous maternity providers, including physician Philip Burgin, echo it:

You have to almost prove to me that you can have a successful vaginal delivery. And it used to be the reverse. We used to get grilled on our cases as residents as to why you did a c-section, and they would analyze it in nau-seating detail. Could you have done something different? Did you have to do it then? Could you have waited? . . . You had to defend yourself if you did one . . . and so it presented to us . . . that this was something to be avoided, that the vaginal delivery is what you should do at all cost. Now I think it's the other way around.

In other words, hospitals pass messages along to maternity providers in grand rounds and in peer reviews that the c-section rate is not used as a measure of quality care. These meetings are ways that hospitals can di-rect care and communicate concern about malpractice. Part of this is ac-complished by *not* using the c-section rate as a quality measure, a sort of sweeping-under-the-rug movement of c-sections as an important outcome to minimize.

The Rule Makers: Organizations

The protocols that guide care are not drawn out of thin air. They are guided by organizations. There is usually a hospital committee that makes these policies, although the structure of the committee varies among hospitals. There will always be a clinical presence—doctors and nurses—and they have strong input from hospital administrators, usually from the risk man-agement department. ACOG recommendations play strongly in hospital policies, but local experience or results of quality assurance data also are included (e.g., lawsuits, complication rates, "near miss" reports of mistakes made in patient care) and may make protocols even stricter than ACOG recommendations.

Maternity providers told me that hospital administrators have a strong hand in developing and implementing protocols. Physician Jack Bianco tells me, "You have your own risk management looking at how to mini-mize things. But what that comes down to is doing more c-sections, still doing more c-sections." Physician Christopher Froehlich concurs: "We are much more actively managing risk. Risk management is a big part of hos-pital care now for maternity as well as medical patients, surgical patients, and that's a change from twenty years ago, and insurance companies have a large part to do with that." Physician Froehlich makes clear the levels of organizational control over protocols. Hospitals set policies, sometimes in reaction to lawsuits, and sometimes because their malpractice insurance company tells them the hospital will not be covered if certain protocols are not followed. As Bill Barth, chair of the ACOG Practice Committee, tells me, "There are a lot of policies out there. Hospitals, regional hospital systems, universities, or third-party payers can come up with all kinds of requirements, or insurers."

Further, documentation becomes important, something I explored in chapter 1. It is not enough for maternity providers to simply follow protocols. They must also *document* that they have followed protocols, hence their preoccupation with documentation. The common wisdom is that if they do not document what they are doing, it is as if they have not done it. Maternity providers focus on documenting that they followed protocols— doing so may protect them from liability in the case of a bad outcome. Studies have found when patient safety protocols are initiated, documentation increases, which helps to explain why I so commonly heard about documentation pressures in my interviews.[55]

Conclusion

Protocols then can be seen as control structures used to constrain the actions and decisions of organizational actors; yet they are not based on sound scientific evidence, and they lead to more and more c-sections. When protocols are followed, policies are adhered to, and guidelines are abided by, any bad outcome will be defined as "maloccurrence," not as "malpractice." In other words, the bad outcome will *not* be attributed to a medical error *because* maternity providers followed the "rules." This truth becomes quite precarious when one realizes that many negative birth outcomes will occur regardless of care. But the care a woman receives, in terms of strict following of the accepted standard of care, will allow a maternity provider to say, "It wasn't my fault," even when following the protocols did not prevent the bad outcome and *not* following the protocols would not have *caused* the bad outcome. The rules reign supreme and become the overriding focus of maternity providers and hospital administrators. Ironically, although all the actors involved want perfect birth outcomes, following the "rules" in some cases will not ensure a good birth outcome and deviating from the "rules" might help a woman to attain a vaginal birth.

The patient safety movement has exacerbated these effects by focusing on standardization, common language, collaboration, and jettisoning c-section rates as quality measures. Combined, as I have discussed in this chapter, they contribute to the c-section rate increase. In fact, I suggest that the patient safety movement in obstetrics is harming women in the name of safety because it perpetuates practices and protocols that lead to more and more c-sections.

Perhaps most concerning is the link that is made in the literature between the patient safety movement and reducing malpractice claims. There is no doubt that it would be good to make birth safer for *women and children*. But, by linking patient safety to preventing malpractice claims, the focus inevitably is on eliminating risk to the baby, not to the mother, because providers perceive that lawsuits are filed for fetal death or injury, not injury to the woman. If the focus were on preventing risk to the woman, part of the patient safety initiative would, no doubt, be on reducing the c-section rate. But ensuring quality of care for women is not on the patient safety radar screen.

A welcome exception to this dominant movement is the California Maternal Quality Care Collaborative, a state-funded agency that focuses on measures of maternal care and uses evidence-based research to suggest ways to improve maternal care, including a focus on reducing the c-section rate. This organization stands out for its concerted effort to improve women's maternal health outcomes, but too few states exhibit this focus on maternal health. California is clearly a leader on this front.

It is more typical in the patient safety movement for c-section rates to be considered "additional measures" in the studies *because* c-section rate is *not* defined as a quality measure in this movement. One study claims proudly that when the authors initiated patient safety initiatives their c-section rate increased by only 1 percent, from 39 percent to 40 percent, not a significant change.[56] They suggested that this is laudable even though the rate is well above the national average and much higher than benchmarks set for optimal women's health. This is further evidence that the c-section rate is not on the radar screen of the patient safety movement. These protocol imperatives tied to the patient safety movement make c-sections more, rather than less, appealing.

Let me conclude by returning to the analogy to the airline industry that I discussed at the beginning of the chapter: "Standardized emergency checklists, simulation training in the conduct of emergencies, uniform policies for the conduct of normal flight operations, extensive review of adverse outcomes." This is a common analogy used in the patient safety literature to advocate for standardization, but it strikes me as misplaced in birth, where different paths may all be normal and result in a positive birth outcome. There is no one best way to birth, and insisting on standardization may have deleterious effects. As I mentioned at the beginning of the chapter, the emphasis on safety may be more relevant in other units of the hospital, but the safest thing in labor and birth is usually less intervention and individualized care. Further, in birth, good outcomes cannot be guaranteed by strictly following protocols. There are no wrong limbs to operate on or wrong-site surgeries to be had in labor and birth, and most preventable adverse obstetrical outcomes are a *result* of interventions and c-sections. Thus birth outcomes are not likely to be improved with this focus on safety as it has been defined in the patient safety movement because this movement has a hand in the increasing c-section rate.

3

Too Much Information

How Technology Raises the Stakes

Unfortunately, some aspects of medicine have become more technological, trying to get [there] before something bad happens. . . . Doctors try to do everything . . . evidence-based. . . . But the few evidence-based medical [studies are] still passed over by this fear that I'm going to be sued. So the [low] threshold of going to c-section—just because it's so available, it's so well developed, and we're checking every single little thing—has made the c-section rate higher.

—Physician Geneva Spalding

Physician Spalding tells me this during our meeting in a basement office of her busy urban practice. Doctor Spalding is upbeat, friendly, and, of the physicians I interviewed, one of the least anxious about liability risk. She has a very go-with-the-flow attitude as she jubilantly greets me, shows me pictures of her children, and assures me that my late arrival because of a forgotten audio recorder is not a problem. "Don't worry! Don't worry!" she tells me. Yet, even with this seemingly unflappable attitude, she tells me how maternity providers use technology not only to avert the occurrence of a bad birth outcome, but even more so to diminish the *liability risk* of a bad outcome. Linking the use of technology to liability risk and c-sections is a rather big leap to make, and I will demonstrate in this chapter how the leap is real and compelling. This chapter examines how organizations negotiate uncertain economic, political, and legal environments at least partly through defining how technology should be used, particularly in a quest to avoid blame for a bad outcome.

The decisions about what technology to use in labor and birth occur over time and happen in medical practices and in hospitals. ACOG is a leader in defining the appropriate use of technology, but just as hospitals sometimes have more restrictive protocols than ACOG advises, sometimes practices and hospitals also develop stricter uses of technology. The fact that most technologies used routinely in labor and birth do not improve outcomes is evidence that their use is tied to other goals. Midwife Candace Whitt tells me there is likely a divergence between what women think and what maternity providers know technology does. She tells me, "The other thing that would be shocking is [to] ask . . . women, . . . 'Do you think that technology has improved mortality and morbidity of our babies over the past thirty years?' And I think every provider would say to you, 'No,' and every woman would say, 'Yes.' . . . There's a dichotomy." This chapter explores that tension.

Prevalence of Technology

Women who give birth in hospitals will all be exposed to technology, at the very least technology to monitor the baby's heart rate and the woman's blood pressure. However, the technologies used are usually far more numerous than just these two. In fact, women may find that technologies used in labor and birth look a bit like a conveyor belt in a factory, which may be why they are commonly referred to as "a cascade of interventions."[1] Women may jump or be pushed onto this conveyer belt at a number of points, but once they're on it, they may find it hard to get off until they come to the end of the process—birth. Induction, augmentation, continuous monitoring, analgesic pain relief—any of these can be the start of a cascade of interventions, sometimes ending in c-section. This conveyor-belt-like experience is something I heard repeatedly in the interviews of women. For example, Cecelia, a woman who gave birth vaginally after a scheduled induction, began to question the interventions she received:

> I'm like, "I don't know how long this is going to go for," but I couldn't handle [the pain] [so I asked for an epidural]. . . . [Then] her heart rate was going down with these Mount Everest [contractions]. . . . I didn't know it was serious until we had two nurses and a doctor and someone else come in and be like, "OK, well, the baby's not really responding that well." . . . They came in and gave me an oxygen mask, which was horrible. I felt like I couldn't breathe, and my mouth was dry, and I was freaking out. I started getting nauseous, and I had the shakes. I had to rip the mask off to throw up. At that point, then my husband started asking questions about what does this mean . . . because I had been telling him, once you start with one

intervention, it's sort of this big domino effect—these movies and books will tell you. He was getting worried, too, that we were going to have to do a c-section, seeing as how much I was really trying to avoid it.

From having her labor artificially started, to her baby's heartbeat being continuously monitored with CTG, to having to breathe through an oxygen mask, these are all technologies used often in the domino-effect way described by Cecelia.[2]

Ultrasounds

Let me begin with an examination of ultrasound technology, which has been introduced into nearly every pregnancy in the United States.[3] Ultrasounds are high-frequency sound waves that produce two- or three-dimensional images, allowing visualization of the baby.[4] Ultrasound is commonly used toward the end of a woman's pregnancy to predict the baby's weight as a way of searching for "large" babies. Shoulder dystocia is more likely to occur with large, or macrosomic, babies, typically defined as babies weighing over 4,500 grams (9 pounds, 15 ounces), which is the reason that maternity providers search for large babies. The likelihood of shoulder dystocia is highest for macrosomic babies; however, because the number of macrosomic babies born is small, half of all cases of shoulder dystocia actually occur in babies who weigh less than 4,000 grams (8 pounds, 13 ounces) at birth.[5] Because of the fear of shoulder dystocia, maternity providers sometimes recommend delivering babies by scheduled c-section if the baby is predicted to weigh over 4,500 grams. This is a concerning practice because the incidence of shoulder dystocia does not decrease when suspected macrosomic babies are delivered by prophylactic c-section.[6]

Let me explain more about shoulder dystocia so it is clearer why ultrasound and prophylactic c-section do not reduce the incidence of the condition. Recall from the introduction that shoulder dystocia is an unpredictable event and happens when a baby's head is delivered but her shoulders get caught behind the woman's pubic bone. Shoulder dystocia may result in a clavicular or brachial plexus injury, and at the most extreme, the baby may die due to lack of oxygen. Shoulder dystocia occurs infrequently. The incidence ranges from 0.2 percent to 3 percent of all vaginal births, with this large range being due to the subjective nature of defining shoulder dystocia.[7] Brachial plexus injuries are quite rare and occur in 0.15 percent of all births.[8] Even more rare is for the brachial plexus injury to be permanent. Only 10 percent of cases of shoulder dystocia result in a permanent injury to the brachial plexus nerve.[9] It is also important to understand that not all brachial plexus injuries are due to shoulder dystocia. Such injuries can occur in utero or during any birth because the baby's neck can be stretched. In fact, nearly half of all brachial plexus injuries occur in births in which there is *not* shoulder dystocia, and most cases of shoulder dystocia do *not* result in brachial plexus injury.[10] This explains why the rate of brachial plexus injuries has remained constant over the past decade, even as the c-section rate has soared.[11]

Let me put the risk of brachial plexus injury into context by comparing the risk of brachial plexus injury to a child's risk of injury from riding in an automobile. The risk of a child under the age of fifteen suffering an injury in an automobile accident is 0.28 percent, about twice the risk of a brachial plexus injury at birth (0.15 percent).[12] Yet we don't typically forbid our children from riding in cars in order to prevent them from being in an accident. When they ride in cars, we don't constantly worry about the risk of an accident. We don't say to ourselves when we arrive safely at the grocery store with a child in tow, "Whew! It was sure lucky we weren't in an automobile accident!" We assume we will arrive safely. My point is that the risk of brachial plexus injuries is viewed much more seriously than are the normal risks children face in our society.

Even if babies predicted to be big by ultrasound aren't scheduled for a c-section delivery, just having an ultrasound toward the end of pregnancy increases a woman's risk of c-section regardless of how big the baby is predicted to be. Specifically, researchers have found that women who have an ultrasound performed in the last month of pregnancy are 44 percent more likely to have a c-section than are women who do not have an ultrasound in the last month of pregnancy, and this increased risk goes up to 85 percent for women whose babies are estimated to weigh over 3,500 grams (7 pounds, 11 ounces).[13] Importantly, the researchers took out the effects of, or controlled for, the baby's birth weight; maternal factors, such as age, race, and obesity; and whether the labor was induced.[14] Further, babies who have an ultrasound-predicted weight over 4,500 grams (9 pounds, 15 ounces) are more likely to be delivered by c-section than are babies whose ultrasound-predicted weight is less than 4,000 grams (8 pounds, 13 ounces), controlling for the baby's actual weight at birth.[15] In other words, the baby's predicted weight, *not* the baby's actual weight, increases the likelihood of c-section. In short, this research suggests an important effect of ultrasound on clinical practice when maternity providers believe a baby may be big—they jump more quickly to a c-section. Importantly, they have this information only because an ultrasound was performed. Twelve percent of primary (or first) c-sections are done because of a suspected "big baby."[16]

Leaving aside the problem with maternity providers' fearing large babies when the vaginal birth of most large babies is not marked by shoulder dystocia, a glaring technical problem exists with the practice of searching for large babies via ultrasound: ultrasound technology is neither a reliable nor a precise predictor of a baby's weight, particularly in the last trimester, when the ultrasound prediction of a baby's weight can be plus or minus 16–20 percent of the actual birth weight.[17] Further, this error of variability is greatest for macrosomic babies.[18] "They told me he was going to be eight pounds, eight to ten pounds, and he's six pounds. Little. I'm like, what? I'm expecting him to be so [big], and he can't fit into . . . his clothes," says Sabrina, a twenty-year-old woman who gave birth vaginally. This is a common refrain from women who were told they were having "big" babies. In fact, it is because of this large error of prediction that ACOG does *not* recommend using ultrasound alone to predict the occurrence of macrosomia.[19] In fact medical researchers Melamed and colleagues, in a 2010 study published in the *Journal of Ultrasound in Medicine*, suggest that the c-section rate could be reduced by as much as 5 percent if an ultrasound technology were developed that had a lower false positive rate (i.e., is less likely to predict that an average-weight baby is macrosomic).[20]

In short, there is no way to reliably predict the birth weight of a baby or the occurrence of shoulder dystocia. Still, it was a common theme in my interviews for maternity providers to speak about searching for "big babies" with ultrasound and delivering them by c-section as a way to avoid the legal risk of a bad outcome. Here physician Leticia Stites describes this practice:

> To prevent one shoulder dystocia that might happen very rarely and is completely unpredictable, you're going to do a lot of c-sections because the baby might be too big. . . . You're doing a lot of unnecessary c-sections to prevent the possibility of one unknown complication that might happen in, I don't know, a thousand or ten thousand cases. It's ridiculous. But you have to do it because if you don't and something bad happens, you're really in trouble.

The trouble to which Doctor Stites refers is a malpractice lawsuit. Her concern is that she will be blamed for shoulder dystocia if the baby is big. It is clear how her decision making is affected by the structure of medical care and the legal system, which drive her use of technology in a quest to prevent being blamed for a bad outcome.

Ultrasound technology also may detect conditions used to justify c-sections, and it is common for women to have multiple ultrasounds in their pregnancies, thereby increasing the likelihood that such a condition will be found.[21] Nurse Diana Ainsworth notes this practice:

> We are seeing into the womb like we never saw before. So we are doing level two, level three ultrasounds on these women. We're finding whether it's an imperfection in the placenta, or this or that, and so it's deemed a high-risk pregnancy, so they don't want to risk anything. . . . The increasing technology supposedly is predicting trouble down the road, so they just go for a c-section.

The practice of using ultrasounds to try to find "large" babies and other "risky" conditions may help to explain why routine ultrasound screens in late pregnancy do not confer any maternal or fetal benefit but instead increase a woman's chance of having a c-section.[22] This heightened surveillance leads to a sense of inevitable risk of vaginal birth.

Induction of Labor

Recall that 41 percent of pregnant women in the United States and in our sample have their labors artificially started.[23] Labor induction is not risk free. Drugs used for induction can overstimulate the uterus and cause it to contract too strongly or too quickly (a condition called tachysystole), which can lead to fetal distress and, at the extreme, uterine rupture and fetal death.[24] Another possible risk of induction occurs when Cytotec is used to ripen a woman's cervix, an "off-label" use of the drug because it is not approved for obstetrical use. Even more worrisome is that Cytotec has been anecdotally linked to increased risk of uterine rupture and maternal death. These reports are concerning enough that *Cochrane Review* researchers have called for maternity providers to report such incidents so that they do not slip through reporting cracks.[25] It's important to note here that the use of Cytotec, which may be harmful to women, is an indication that risk to the mother's life is not as important as risk to the baby's life. This is likely driven by hospital administrators' and maternity providers' perceptions that lawsuits are filed for the death and injury of babies rather than of women, a topic I explore more in chapter 5.

Induction also increases a woman's chance of having a c-section. Women whose labors are induced are twice as likely to have a c-section as those women who begin labor spontaneously.[26] This was also the case in the sample of women we studied. Of the women who attempted a vaginal birth, 23 percent of women who were induced had a c-section compared to 12 percent of women who were not induced. Women who have not given birth before and are induced when the cervix is closed have a very high chance of having a c-section. These women have an astounding 50 percent c-section rate—that is, a one-in-two chance of having a c-section.[27]

Further, it is important to note that Pitocin is used commonly to augment a woman's labor, regardless of whether she is induced, and use of Pitocin increases a woman's risk of c-section by about 15 percent.[28] In our sample, over 50 percent of women who attempted a vaginal birth received Pitocin, although their c-section rates were not that different—18.2 percent of women who received Pitocin and 17.6 percent of women who didn't receive Pitocin had a c-section.

Women are induced for a variety of reasons. Sometimes the inductions are considered to be medically indicated—being overdue, having a maternal health problem that requires an early birth, or having a concern with the baby's health or with the baby's becoming "too big." At other times the induction has no medical indication. For example, the woman wants to control the day the baby is born or who will deliver the baby, or the woman is anxious for the baby to be born or to be through with pregnancy. A maternity provider may also recommend induction for a nonmedical reason such as to deliver a woman before he or she takes a planned vacation. Nonmedically indicated inductions are commonly referred to as "social inductions."

The line between social inductions and medical inductions is exceptionally blurry. Just as delivering suspected macrosomic babies by prophylactic c-section has not been shown to decrease the risk of shoulder dystocia or to improve fetal outcomes, there also is no evidence that inducing the labors of women who have suspected "big" babies before their due dates improves outcomes.[29] Yet, having a suspected big baby is commonly considered a medical indication for induction. In fact, the fear of shoulder dystocia occurring in the births of big babies leads to policies where physicians induce nearly all women who have diabetes mellitus or gestational diabetes and most women with suspected macrosomic babies before their due dates, a practice not grounded in empirical evidence of improved outcomes.[30] I heard this commonly from maternity providers like physician Molly Nichols, who tells me, "We're getting more . . . patients who are diagnosed with diabetes, who are having these larger babies. . . . Sometimes we induce them because of the diabetes." Similar to the worry they have about delivering a big baby vaginally, providers worry that babies of diabetic women will have shoulder dystocia and that the medical staff will be blamed if this happens. Thus the providers suggest induction before a woman's due date to prevent the baby from growing "too big."

We interviewed eight women who identified themselves as having been diagnosed with gestational diabetes or diabetes mellitus and who planned a vaginal birth, and all but one were induced before forty weeks gestation. As Jacqueline, a twenty-nine-year-old woman who had a vaginal birth, says, "I was induced . . . because I had gestational diabetes. So I *had to be induced.*" Likewise, Roxanne was induced because she had gestational diabetes and her physician did not want the baby to grow "too big." Roxanne did not want to be induced because she had heard that inductions were painful and because she wished to avoid interventions, including pain relief and a c-section. But, because she was told that it was in her baby's best interest, she decided in favor of induction. All of her plans went astray. Not only was she induced and had an epidural, she also had an emergency c-section for failure to progress in labor. Four other women were induced because maternity providers feared their babies would be too big. Some women realize afterward that the induction may not have been necessary. Anya tells us, "Because he isn't as big as I thought he was, maybe I should have just waited and not chosen to do an induction."

Other women shared stories of "soft" medical reasons for induction, in the following case for swollen feet and legs. This induction ended in an emergency c-section:

> I had a lot of swelling and issues with my feet and legs, so my doctor wanted me to be induced. . . . I came in at ten o'clock . . . and then started Pitocin at one o'clock, and I was in labor until about nine thirty [the next day]. And then her head was just too big. It wasn't going to fit, and then also the epidural wasn't working on my left side so I was in a lot of pain; I was feeling all of my contractions. . . . The anesthesiologist said that if I rolled over on my left side, they could give me more medicine . . . but

when I did that, her heart rate would drastically drop down, so then they started freaking out about that. . . . They had me go in for a c-section . . . That was really scary because that was the one thing that I did not want to have happen. (Jessica)

While we can debate whether inducing women diagnosed with diabetes or who have severe swelling is medically indicated, some inductions are clearly done with no medical indication. These social inductions are often encouraged by maternity providers—or if not encouraged, at least tolerated. Social inductions are done for a number of reasons, some which are tied to women's needs or desires. In terms of the LTMII survey, of those women who were induced, 27 percent said the induction was for a non-medical reason such as controlling the timing of the birth or wanting to be done with the pregnancy.[31] Interestingly, none of the women we interviewed indicated either of these reasons for the induction, although, of course, there may be social pressures not to disclose such reasons to an interviewer. In contrast, care providers suggested that pregnant women often choose social inductions. Nurses spoke to me more than physicians did about their perception of women being socially induced. It may be that women are more upfront with nurses about why they are being induced, or it may be that physicians are loathe to admit that they induce women for nonmedical reasons. Nurse Margie Napolitano tells me:

I see people [being induced] because it's the first day of school and they want to be home for their other child. I see people do it because it's Christmas and they want to be home for Christmas. People do it because their husband is going out of town on a business trip and they want to be induced now. People do it because they are sick of being pregnant and they just want the baby out.

Another reason for induction that I heard about from physicians and nurses is that women may try to control which of the physicians in the practice will deliver their babies. With the spread of large practices, doctors rotate call, and women play a game of chance with who will be the doctor on call if they wait to arrive at the hospital in spontaneous labor—will it be the doctor they love or the doctor they hate or the doctor they have never met? As physician Philip Burgin tells me, "We tell everybody right up front that we are a group practice, . . . where all the patients are all of our patients. So if we have a doctor on call, that's the doctor who will do the delivery on that day, regardless of [who] you saw first in the practice." Scheduling an induction can help women to avoid the problem of not knowing who will be at the birth. National survey data suggest that of the women who are induced, 8 percent gave this as a reason.[32] We did not hear this from any of the women we interviewed, although maternity providers say they commonly see it. Nurse April Colman tells me, "Oftentimes they do [want to be induced] because you have a group of six physicians and there's two you click with and four you don't." This becomes a more prevalent problem as large practices continue to grow. Sometimes inductions may also be tied to a physician's personal vacation schedule. Midwife Erika Soule says, "I've seen women asking their doctors when they're going to be on vacation, and if . . . their due date is right around when they leave, they might talk about possibly being induced."

These are common reasons for social inductions, and notice how maternity providers perceive the reasons to be driven by women's choices. However, I would argue that the organization of the medical profession has constrained women's choices. For example, with the growth of large practices, women are not guaranteed continuity of care but must jockey for having the physician they prefer deliver their babies. Women's choices are constrained, too, by the lack of social support for families, such that women are worried about who will watch their other children during the birth and about the inflexibility of employers around the uncertainty of the timing of childbirth. Further, there are just as many reasons to socially induce a woman that are not tied to what women want, but rather to the maternity provider's interests and desires. I heard often that inductions are convenient for maternity providers. For example, physician Lawrence Rascon tells me, "A doctor is in his office, he does things—maybe he tried to induce someone who may not be the best candidate for induction because he's going to be off that week." Nurse Anne Conaway also worries about this:

> There's always that little bitty part of me who wonders how much it is for the convenience of the doctor—"I won't have to go in the middle of the night if I induce my patient" and "Christmas is coming and I've got these five patients and if I induce them all for post dates before the holiday maybe I won't have to go in on Christmas day."

There is also a liability overlay to induction, especially when women are induced to prevent them from delivering past their due dates. Maternity providers worry that if they don't induce women by their due dates and there is a bad outcome, they will be blamed for allowing the pregnancy to continue "too long." It is important to note that the definition of being "over due" has changed over time.[33] The "normal" pregnancy length is defined as a four-week window between thirty-eight and forty-two weeks since the start of the woman's last menstrual period (a woman's "due date" is in the middle of this window, at forty weeks), and, if allowed, some women's pregnancies will go beyond forty-two weeks. However, maternity providers latch on to the due date as important because empirical research finds a slight elevation in stillbirths in women whose pregnancies extend beyond forty-one weeks. The risk is considered quite rare, and the number of stillbirths is too low to draw a statistical finding distinguishing outcomes for women induced at forty or forty-one weeks and outcomes for women who continue their pregnancies through forty-two weeks.[34] *Cochrane Review* researchers indicate that women should be "appropriately counseled on both the relative and absolute risk" of continuing a pregnancy beyond forty-one weeks.[35] Yet the fear of stillbirth drives the practice of inducing women earlier and earlier. In fact, the average gestational age in the United States is decreasing. The most common length of gestation in the United States has dropped from forty weeks to thirty-nine weeks and the proportion of births that occur after forty weeks gestation has declined while earlier-than-terms births in the thirty-seven- to thirty-nine-week gestation range have increased.[36] In fact, a woman's being "overdue" was the most common reason for induction in the LTMII survey and also among the women we interviewed.[37] Only one woman out of the eighty-three women who we interviewed, or 1.2 percent of women we interviewed, gave birth after forty-one weeks gestation.

This trend is important because induction increases a woman's risk of having a c-section. Yet women are typically induced before forty-one weeks regardless of this risk because obstetrical practices sometimes make this a mandatory policy, as described by physician Philip Burgin:

We're currently evaluating whether we're going to start doing forty-one-week inductions or not. . . . [It's] not because we think we'll get better results. [It's] because everybody who gives lectures on this—guys from Yale . . . and [the University of Connecticut]—say you should be doing it at forty-one weeks. Even though ACOG doesn't say that, they say it. So these are going to be the expert witnesses against us. Who are you going to get to be the expert witness for you? . . . They'll get somebody like me, an average Joe, who will come in and say, "Yeah, this is how I do it." But they won't have the weight of the guy from Yale or [the University of Connecticut]. So we will probably be changing this policy very soon. . . . This is completely malpractice driven—this decision—completely malpractice driven.

Physician Philip Burgin gives insight into how practices may develop induction policies guided almost solely by liability concerns that push the average gestation age at birth earlier and earlier.

The liability concern extends beyond due dates. Women are sometimes induced when anything unusual shows up in prenatal testing. As physician Lawrence Rascon tells me, the heightened vigilance in prenatal care leads to inductions because of the overlay of concern with liability risk:

When we do some anti-partum testing on the patient, any little thing that shows the baby may have a problem, we're more likely to induce those people. . . . You don't want to send a patient home who may have a funny strip on the monitor because if you send the mother home [and] the baby dies, you're dead. So you're more likely to keep that patient. Say the mother comes in and says the baby's not moving that much. And she's forty weeks, let's say. And you see a little blip on the monitor that doesn't look quite right, but it's probably OK. You're less likely to send that mother home and say, "OK, let's wait until labor comes on." You're more likely to say, "You know what, we've got to get you induced because this baby may have a problem." And so those are people who have much higher chances of a section because their cervix isn't quite ready yet.

Melissa, a thirty-two-year-old woman who planned a vaginal birth but had an emergency c-section following a failed induction, has a story that bears a striking resemblance to Doctor Rascon's warning:

My . . . OB stripped my membranes at the appointment; I was thirty-nine and a half weeks. . . . This is my second boy, and I was early with the first one, so they were just assuming that I'd be early again. So, then I had contractions [every] five minutes, but they weren't very strong, so I took my time and stayed home through the night and ended up coming to the hospital at ten in the morning the next day. . . . Nothing was really happening . . . but the baby's heart rate was too slow so they kept me here . . . for about four or five hours, and then they finally admitted us and induced me . . . and that increased my contractions, the severity and the frequency, but [it was] not really dilating me. I got up to about four centimeters, and they decided to break my water. . . . I asked for an epidural. . . . Then my contractions were really strong and furious, and they determined that the baby's heart rate was just too variable and got too many dips, and I ended up having to do an emergency cesarean.

It is important to understand that we cannot make a clinical assessment of Melissa from her story. But her story is illustrative of women who, despite seemingly little clinical risk, have birth experiences that escalate from induction to c-section.

Epidurals

Most women have analgesic pain relief during labor—only 14 percent of women do not use pain medication.[38] Recall that epidural analgesic is the most common form of medical pain relief—71 percent of women receive an epidural during labor. Twenty-two percent of women use narcotic pain relief such as Demerol or Stadol, and the vast majority of the women who use narcotics also receive an epidural—16 percent of women receive both.[39] Epidural use was very common in the sample of women we interviewed; 86 percent of women who attempted a vaginal birth received an epidural. Epidurals are not risk free. They are associated with side effects such as reduced maternal blood pressure (hypotension), itchiness, drowsiness, shivering, and maternal fever.[40] Rare but severe side effects, such as debilitating headaches, can also result if the dura, which encloses the spinal cord and spinal fluid, is accidently punctured.[41] Epidurals also increase the risk of other interventions, such as Pitocin (because epidurals often slow down labor), catheterization (because women are not able to feel their legs to walk to the toilet), and instrumental delivery (because women may not be able to feel in order to push).[42] Women who receive epidurals are also more likely to have a c-section for fetal distress than are women who do not have an epidural.[43] Further, research finds that epidurals teamed with low-dose Pitocin augmentation increase a woman's chance of having a c-section.[44]

It is also important to understand that epidurals increase the length of the second stage of labor (pushing the baby out).[45] Anything that increases the second stage of labor allows the image of shoulder dystocia to form in the minds of maternity providers. As midwife Rosalie Batten tells me, when a woman is suspected of having a big baby and she has a long second stage of labor, maternity providers' concern with shoulder dystocia is palpable: "Babies in your mind get bigger and bigger the longer the labor goes on. 'Oh my God, that baby, it was nine pounds, but it's eleven [pounds] now.'" In short, as Batten tells me, "When women are slower than we think [they ought to be], it is time to do a c-section." Thus an epidural can indirectly lead to a c-section if the provider develops a concern about shoulder dystocia due to the woman's decreased ability to push.

Part of the reason for such a high epidural rate is due to an unintended consequence of the focus on documentation. In popular culture, it is believed that the use of epidurals is tied to women's fear of pain and desire to be medicated. This is sometimes the case. For example, in response to the question "During your pregnancy, did you have an expectation or a wish about what your labor and birth would be like?" we commonly heard answers like "I was hoping it would be as painless as possible," "Pain free," and "I don't like pain. I'm really, really bad with pain." But it is not just that women fear pain, it is also that they are not given many options to deal with pain other than medication and are typically tethered to the bed by the use of continuous CTG. Further, maternity providers do not always expect women can handle labor pain without medication. Midwives commonly told me that nurses have a general discomfort with unmedicated women. But there are good reasons for nurses to want a calm labor and delivery unit. Nurses must spend their time documenting, and paperwork is hard to complete if they have two unmedicated patients and need to help both of them through labor and birth, as articulated by nurse Jane Rios:

> [Nurses] become dependent upon epidurals as well because natural childbirth when you're in the hospital is hard. I mean women are uncomfortable. It means rubbing their back, it means helping them squat, showers. It means a lot more hands-on. And . . . today you're having a lot more paperwork. . . . You actually enjoy the patient who is lying there in the bed, calm, relaxed, watching TV, and napping, and you can catch up on your notes or whatever. . . . From the nursing perspective, it can be very accommodating for them to have an epidural so you can get your work done.

In fact, many women told us that they were pressured to receive epidurals. Yet this overreliance on epidurals may point women toward c-sections.

Monitoring the Fetal Heart Rate Continuously

Beyond the artificial starting and pacing of labor and the use of pain medications, another part of labor management, which I've explored in earlier chapters, is the monitoring of the fetal heart rate and uterine contraction patterns during labor. Continuous cardiotocography (CTG) is used almost universally in hospitals in the United States to monitor the fetal heart pattern.[46] CTG is the most common obstetric procedure in the United States.[47] Its use has grown over the years from 44.6 percent in 1980 to 62.2 percent in 1988 to nearly 100 percent by 2005.[48] I focus here on how the use of CTG has increased at the same time that other technologies to help interpret the CTG strip have gone by the wayside.

Recall that there is no evidence that the use of continuous CTG decreases the likelihood of neurological disease, such as cerebral palsy, or fetal death, and the false positive rate of continuous CTG is as high as 99.8 percent, which means that 99.8 percent of babies identified to have non-reassuring heart rate patterns by CTG will not be compromised at birth.[49] Stated differently, "Almost every positive test result is wrong."[50] It is the lack of predictability of electronic fetal monitors and their unfettered use that lead providers to intervene quickly when babies have "non-reassuring" fetal heart rate patterns. The baby with a non-reassuring fetal heart rate pattern could be in the 0.2 percent of babies who are actually compromised.

Physician Lawrence Rascon talks about this perceived risk: "You'd have to do a lot of sections to avoid the one baby. . . . When we're looking at a baby in real time on the monitor during the mother's labor and things don't look so good, we don't know which one it is. They all look the same." Nurses are very aware of this high false positive rate. Nurse Michele Saxton tells me, "Because we don't really know when . . . the baby is oxygenating well, you tend to move toward c-section a lot sooner. And, I tell you, nine times out of ten, you take that baby out, and it's pink and screaming and perfectly fine." Likewise, Physician Joe Haley says, "So, if you say, 'Oh my God! I've got to do a cesarean section because the strip doesn't look good,' you're going to be wrong approximately 98 to 99 percent of the time. The baby is going to be fine. . . . But, if you don't do it [and there is a bad outcome] . . . then you're going to be faulted."

This error of the technology could be averted completely by monitoring the labor of low-risk women with intermittent auscultation (checking the baby's heart rate intermittently with a handheld Doppler unit), which does not pick up as many worrisome decelerations as continuous CTG but has fetal outcomes just as good as continuous CTG.[51] But maternity providers have learned that the physical evidence provided by the fetal monitoring strips is essential if they are to defend themselves against malpractice in the case of a bad birth outcome:

> The guidelines are that people can do intermittent tracing if they want, unless the baby is having issues. There is a protocol to it. By and large, though, [most women] have continuous heart rate monitoring. . . . That, I think, is a good example . . . of trying to protect yourself so that you don't get sued. (Physician Rosemary Steel)

As physician Steel indicates, maternity providers are *highly* critical of the routine use of continuous CTG. They know its use does not improve birth outcomes and that it leads to a higher c-section rate. But they believe that in the current uncertain legal environment, they must have a patient continuously monitored to demonstrate that they are appropriately watching and treating the patient.

Further, intermittent auscultation is not used because, according to ACOG guidelines, only low-risk women are eligible for the practice.[52] Low-risk patients are those patients in spontaneous labor, with a singleton pregnancy in a head-down position, who have no labor augmentation, pain medication, or previous c-section. Of the sixty-five women we interviewed who attempted a vaginal birth, 40 percent were induced, 86 percent had an epidural, and 51 percent were given Pitocin to augment or induce their labors. On the national level 41 percent of U.S. pregnancies are induced, 71 percent have epidurals, and 55 percent are augmented or induced with Pitocin.[53] Thus few women are "eligible" for intermittent auscultation. Labor and delivery nurse Eva Bunnell describes how unusual it is for her to care for patients defined as "low risk": "They have a reason to be on continuous monitoring, which almost all of our patients are, . . . because most of them are on Pitocin or some sort of inducing. Even if they come in spontaneous labor, a lot of times they end up on Pitocin unless they're really laboring along at an acceptable rate." Thus most women at some point "must" be monitored continuously with CTG to meet ACOG guidelines.

Organizations teach maternity providers how to use technology and how to make decisions using information provided by technology, especially how to monitor CTG strips. I heard from a number of physicians that they learn at conferences how to interpret strips and how strips will be used to fault them. Here physicians Lawrence Rascon and Andrew

Robinette tell me about conferences where they have heard litigating attorneys speak about these topics:

And every time you go to these seminars with obstetrics the first thing they talk about is the malpractice problem. And you keep hearing over and over again, "Protect yourself, protect yourself." We've actually had lecturers come in who are the lawyers [who] sue the doctors . . . and [one] said, "If that monitor strip looks bad for fifteen minutes, if you don't do a section and that baby is dead, you're going to get sued." Now, if you look at monitor strips for pregnant women, you'll have periods the baby doesn't look that good all the time in just about every [case], and most of the babies are fine. So it kind of makes you anxious about every little pregnancy. (Physician Lawrence Rascon)

I can get for you the name of the attorney who gave us this lecture. He's the number one malpractice insurance attorney in New York City. . . . So that's a big deal. And he said to us, "Two decelerations, I got you." (Physician Andrew Robinette)

It seems quite understandable, then, given the lack of reliability of CTG strips and the 99.8 percent false positive rate, that maternity providers are quite fearful of "bad strips." Lawrence Rascon goes on to tell me how lawsuits are based on monitoring strips, even though this measure lacks predictability of a bad birth outcome:

Now we're in a catch-22. Scientifically, if you look at the literature, the monitors have not prevented cerebral palsy, but every single legal case that's brought with a bad baby, they show the monitor. Every case. . . . That's the basis of the case. Because if you have a bad baby and you have a perfect monitor strip, you're not going to get sued because how would you know the baby's bad if you have a perfect monitor?

The catch-22 here is that providers say that nearly all fetal monitoring strips have some kind of "abnormality" in them that could be used to suggest that a c-section should be done. Maternity providers tell me that any time a strip from a bad outcome is reviewed, it is always found to have something wrong with it. As physician Joe Haley tells me, "I've heard a litigator say [that] . . . he can take any fetal monitor strip and make a malpractice case out of it." There is reason for this concern.

Studies suggest that when asked to review strips, maternity providers are more likely to find abnormality in the strip if they know it is tied to a bad birth outcome.[54]

If there remains any doubt that liability concerns are at the bottom of the use of CTG technology, consider the summary of a research article on CTG published in the *American Journal of Obstetrics and Gynecology*, one of obstetrics' flagship publications: "In our opinion one of the most useful aspects of electronic fetal heart rate monitoring is the generation of continuous strips whose normalcy can be used to refute claims of asphyxia and acidosis as a cause for fetal or neonatal damage."[55] Monitors are used to reduce legal risk, not to improve birth outcomes; yet they have been shown to unquestionably increase the c-section rate.[56] This admission is common in the medical literature on CTG.[57]

Yet it is not simply liability concerns that lead to the use of CTG. There are also organizational pressures that push the use of continuous CTG. For example, CTG allows a nurse to monitor more than one patient at a time, meaning that hospitals do not need to have as many nurses on duty. Although there are some hospitals with the luxury of a 1:1 nurse to patient ratio in labor and delivery, that is not standard, and auscultation requires a 1:1 ratio to meet the defined observation periods. It likely makes no difference in fetal outcomes if one monitoring period is missed or if one is done late, but if a baby is born compromised, the missed or late observation may be used as evidence of provider negligence because it is a breech in the standard of care. As physician Lawrence Rascon suggests, hospitals are dependent on electronic fetal monitors because they don't have enough nurses to provide the 1:1 care that would be optimal for intermittent auscultation:

> Now we can't even go back to not [continuously] monitoring for two reasons. One is you couldn't even win a lawsuit if there was no monitoring strip. And the other thing is nursing staff. You couldn't afford to have a nursing staff that big to be 1:1 with every pregnant woman in labor. . . . You need a monitor for personnel things. Because a nurse can watch three monitors at a time with the central monitoring system, . . . you don't need to have a nurse in the room continuously.

The short-staffing issue mentioned by Rascon is particularly important when thinking about monitoring women in labor, because nurses are responsible for monitoring. If a midwife or physician does not want a patient to be continuously monitored, the midwife or physician must stay in the hospital to ensure that this happens. Midwife Rosalie Batten tells me, "When I say this person doesn't need continuous monitoring, the nurse's response is, 'Well, I can't be in that room every 15 minutes . . . to listen to the baby, so if you can do that . . . fine, but otherwise she goes on the monitor.'"

So, while the ease of use of CTG for nurses is often emphasized in common discourse—"It's always there, and you can just watch it from where you are, so it's less labor intensive to just keep them on," nurse Eva Bunnell tells me—there are clearly other reasons for the continuation of its use. Nurses commonly tell me they simply cannot perform auscultation because they have too many patients to monitor and also they must carefully document labor, a time-consuming duty, particularly when hospital administrators make it clear that there is an organizational imperative for meticulous documentation:

> Whether it's actually true or not, there is a perception that intermittent monitoring is more work for [nurses], and I think, too, for them, it makes them feel vulnerable. Because . . . normally they need to document the baseline of the fetal heart rate, what the variability of the heart rate is, whether there are accelerations, whether there are decelerations, and that's not possible with intermittent auscultation. . . . All you can say is what the baseline fetal heart rate was when you listened for that period of time. . . . So, I think that [not having] all this information that is supposed to fit into the slots on their nurse's notes . . . makes them feel nervous. (Midwife Rita Morey)

This is particularly important to understand. Documentation protects maternity providers, and the documentation must be complete. Auscultation does not allow nurses to fill out the charts entirely, making them feel vulnerable for not having total documentation of the labor and birth.

In short, using continuous CTG on nearly all women in labor helps maternity providers and hospital administrators to potentially avert legal risk or defend themselves if a malpractice lawsuit is filed. The use of continuous CTG is also in the hospital's interest because it allows them to hire fewer nurses to monitor women in labor. Further, families are more comfortable because they believe that continuous CTG allows providers to identify babies in trouble. For all of these reasons—not because it improves fetal outcomes—continuous CTG is ubiquitous in American hospitals.

Other Technologies to Monitor the Baby in Labor and Why They Aren't Used

Because it is well understood that CTG is fallible, medical researchers have searched for other tests that can be used to help maternity providers better interpret non-reassuring fetal heart strips. Yet, perhaps not surprisingly given the organizational incentives for maternity providers to use continuous CTG and pay attention to the strips, most of these technologies are not regularly used, leaving the CTG strip to be interpreted in isolation.[58] One of the technologies is to test the pH level of a sample of the baby's blood, taken by scraping the baby's scalp. When a baby is compromised, the acid level of the blood declines; thus the level of pH in a baby's blood indicates how well oxygenated she is. Maternity providers can use this test to reassure themselves in the case of a non-reassuring CTG tracing. However, scalp pH tests are rarely used and, in fact, major manufacturers have stopped selling the kits for a few reasons.[59] First, another now-discarded technology, fetal pulse oximetry, replaced this test.[60] Second, the tests were seen as difficult to perform and costly to maintain, and providers hesitated doing the tests because they left babies' heads scratched, something maternity providers and parents wish to avoid. Most providers told me they have not had access to these tests for years, and none of the eighty-three women we interviewed had such a test performed during her labor.

However, surely a scratch to a baby's scalp is relatively inconsequential if it prevents an unnecessary c-section. Most women we interviewed desired a vaginal birth, and it seems a stretch to believe that they would prefer a c-section over a scratch to the baby's head, particularly when c-sections may result in much more serious fetal lacerations—a small percentage of babies born by c-section are cut during the surgery and suffer permanent scars.[61] Yet, if the risk is presented to women in a way that causes fear that the baby will be damaged, perhaps they will shy away from the test. Notice how physician Jack Bianco talks about the test in the following interview excerpt:

The scalp samples aren't perfect, and they're invasive, and if your baby gets an infection after one of those, they'll sue you for it. Because you didn't tell them, "If I do this to your baby, your baby could get a scalp infection [and] that could lead to your baby's scalp rotting off." Now what are the chances of that happening? It's the chance of some drunk driver running a red light and hitting you on your way home tonight. Not great, but it's pretty dramatic, and if I tell you there is [this risk], you're certainly going to be scared about it. So, here we tell people this could happen, . . . the incidence is anecdotally rare, but because of that, people now don't allow us to do them because they're afraid now their baby will get a problem from it.

Physician Bianco doesn't want to take the risk that the baby will get a scratch. But he is not an unconcerned physician. He is angry that he cannot perform tests that would help to facilitate a vaginal birth.

The interesting thing to note is that maternity providers clearly feel that fetal scalp pH tests allow them to better assess whether a c-section is necessary. Take, for example, the words of physician James Montenegro:

There's been a reduction in our ability [to] reassure ourselves about the fetal well-being of a borderline [CTG] tracing. . . . [In] the past if I had a questionable tracing, didn't know if this baby was OK or not, I was routinely doing . . . scalp pHs. That was taken away from us and replaced by fetal pulse oximetry. . . . I'm going to tell you that there are more c-sections being done now because any questionable tracing gets sectioned. . . . If I had . . . tracings [that were] then and now, I could show you . . . that if I had a reassuring scalp pH, that lady would have had a vaginal delivery. If I had the same tracing without being able to do a scalp pH, she finds herself [with] a c-section.

Physician Montenegro argues that c-sections have increased because maternity providers can no longer be reassured in the face of a questionable CTG strip.

Fetal pulse oximetry is the alternative test to which Doctor Montenegro refers. This technology measures the oxygenation of the baby and is performed by inserting a small catheter into the woman's uterus so that it lies alongside the baby. Tests of this technology suggest that it decreases the likelihood of c-section due to fetal distress but does not have an effect on the overall c-section rate.[62] However, decreasing the likelihood of c-section due to fetal distress is not an insignificant outcome, and studies suggest that a single test of oxygen saturation may reassure physicians that babies are receiving enough oxygen to continue the labor.[63] According to the *Cochrane Review*, "The decision pathway leading to performing a cesarean section may be important. The additional information that fetal pulse oximetry can provide, when a non-reassuring fetal heart rate trace has been identified, may translate to avoidance of a caesarean section for non-reassuring fetal status, with its associated stress levels for the mother and resource implications for the health service providers."[64] As midwife Joyce Linville mentions, the use of pulse oximetry sometime allows labor to continue without rushing to what might be an unnecessary c-section:

> So often you have a tracing that looks terrible, and you go back to c-section and the baby comes out screaming. . . . There should be some other way of testing the test that is reliable. I was so thrilled when the continuous O2 monitoring was being done because it confirmed my suspicion for years that the truth of the matter is [the fetal heart rate] was going up and down, but overall it was probably just fine. And for that brief period of time, I remember just gutsing through, with my attending, tracings that ordinarily we would have gone to section, and the babies were fine.

However, the benefits of fetal pulse oximetry are overshadowed by one study that found that shoulder dystocia risks are higher when pulse oximetry is used.[65] This one study seems to be the basis of ACOG's recommendation against the use of fetal pulse oximetry.[66] The mere threat of an increased risk of shoulder dystocia, though not well established, extinguished the use of pulse oximetry. Because ACOG now recommends against using fetal pulse oximetry to monitor labor, if a negative birth outcome occurs in a birth in which this technology was used, the providers may be accused of negligence because they violated the current standard of care.

Yet another promising technology, electrocardiogram, referred to as ST segment and T wave analysis or STAN, has been used in Europe since the early 1990s to ascertain how the baby is faring in labor. It is typically used when a CTG strip is non-reassuring. STAN allows maternity providers to examine the heart wave patterns as an indication of adequate oxygenation of the baby.[67] STAN technology is rarely used in the United States. When I delved into the reasons for this, I found that the patent is hard to obtain and the cost of staff training and maintenance of the equipment is high. The U.S. National Institutes of Health is currently recruiting participants at thirteen U.S. hospitals for a study examining whether STAN technology has an impact on newborn health, a promising sign for women's and newborns' health, although the adoption of the technology is likely years away.[68] Perhaps the slowness of adoption means that hospital administrators are not interested in implementing costly technology, especially when it is not clear that the technology will increase profits or avert legal risk for a bad outcome. Internationally, STAN is seen as an important technology to help physicians better detects compromised babies. It is supported by randomized trials, something that CTG cannot claim.

The bottom line is that technologies other than continuous CTG are not commonly used to help evaluate the baby's health during labor, and the CTG tracings are often read as "black or white." The fact that CTG is so consistently used in U.S. hospitals even though it has a false positive rate of 99.8 percent speaks to how technology is routinely used in labor and birth to shield maternity providers and hospitals from blame for a bad birth outcome. In short, at least part of the reason for the high c-section rate is that fetal heart rate tracings are typically observed with continuous CTG, and no other tests are used to distinguish when non-reassuring readings are really fine. Recall that according to the LTMII data, 25 percent of primary c-sections are done for a non-reassuring fetal heart beat.

Vacuum and Forceps

Management of labor has changed also in that babies must "drop out"— they are unlikely to be aided by forceps or vacuum extraction, two ways that may facilitate a vaginal birth when a c-section seems inevitable. There is no empirical evidence that a c-section in these cases leads to better outcomes than does instrumental delivery.[69] Forceps have been used, although sometimes too enthusiastically, for the past four hundred years to facilitate vaginal births, and unquestionably may help women avoid a c-section.[70] Comparing countries, it is clear that higher rates of vacuum and forceps delivery are associated with lower c-section rates.[71] Yet few physicians are currently trained in the use of forceps, and even those physicians who are trained in forceps delivery tend to shy away from using them because c-sections are quicker and more predictable and because physicians believe they will be better protected from blame in the case of a bad outcome if the baby is surgically delivered. None of the women we interviewed had a forceps delivery, while 6 percent had a delivery assisted with vacuum extraction. This is consistent with national data suggesting that 7 percent of women have assisted vaginal deliveries.[72] The reluctance of physicians to use forceps and vacuum extraction occurs even among physicians who are trained in these technologies and are confident of their skills, as physician Robert Hinson describes:

The great incentive to do a cesarean again is medical–legal. . . . We don't do forceps or vacuum deliveries. [They] are just becoming history stories in the books. They're just not being done. Not because we don't know how to do them in a good manner, because we've been doing these for twenty years, but because we know that we will blamed for something wrong with the baby if we put a forceps on a baby or a vacuum on a baby, and if we do a cesarean that's considered less traumatic to the baby.

Because forceps, and vacuum to some extent, are rarely used, OB residents receive very little training in the use of these technologies, which causes the withering of their use to proceed ever more quickly, as described by physician Joe Haley:

The other thing about operative deliveries is once you start, if your senior people are hesitant to do this, who is going to train you? . . . The training withers. . . . If you . . . have had experience in [only] one or two [forceps deliveries], they just abandon it as a skill set. . . . It's really an exponential loss of these types of skills and operative deliveries. I've always said in the past [that forceps] are a safe way in general to avoid a cesarean delivery.

Rosemary Steel, who is in her mid-thirties, expresses her reluctance to use forceps: "Forceps for me . . . I just ignore them because I was never trained on them, and I've only seen maybe five cases of them being used."

It seems easier and less risky *to the provider* to perform a c-section. The question that should be asked is whether a c-section is easier and less risky *for the woman* than a forceps or vacuum delivery. Instead, c-sections are performed because maternity providers believe they are better protected from blame in the case of a bad outcome.

Other Organizational Imperatives

Hospitals also have other pressures that influence the use of technology. For example, hospitals increasingly have a shortage of beds in labor and delivery and in postpartum units. Hospitals that were constructed even ten years ago did not build into their construction plans the need to have large postpartum units to allow over one third of women giving birth to stay in the hospital for three or four days. I heard tales of the problem with bed shortages. In one hospital, when postpartum fills up, women are moved to the high-risk floor or stay in labor and delivery, making space in that hospital unit even tighter.

A similar problem occurs because of the increase of *scheduled* c-sections and inductions, which require more beds on certain days and at certain times of the day, specifically between 7:00 a.m. and 5:00 p.m., Monday through Friday. In other words, when birth does not happen spontaneously, there are unnatural ebbs and flows in terms of the number of women in the labor unit at any given time. Maternity providers sometimes report that they need to hurry and get women delivered to clear space for women who are coming in, either in spontaneous labor or for scheduled inductions and c-sections:

> Hospitals, of course, do want patients to come in and go out and to do that in a timely fashion. And on a busy labor and delivery unit, we don't have the luxury of letting moms just kind of hang out. (Physician Rosemary Steel)

This means that augmentation and c-section become more likely because they hasten birth. Labor and birth need to be done quickly to move women along and out of the labor and delivery unit. Again we see how organizational imperatives constrain maternity providers in their practice.

Conclusion

In sum, technologies to start, monitor, and control labor and birth in hospitals, used in an attempt to alleviate liability threats, have led to an ever-higher c-section rate, from ultrasound technology that is used to search for "large" babies to deliver them early, to the artificial beginning and pacing of labor, to the near-universal use of CTG. On the flip side, the technologies that have fallen out of use could prevent c-sections. Fetal pH scalp samples and pulse oximetry may reassure maternity providers of the baby's health when a CTG strip looks worrisome. Even more perplexing is the stalled progress of integrating STAN technology into labor and birth in the United States. This technology, which analyzes the heart waves of babies, has been shown to reduce c-section rates *and* to improve fetal outcomes, but the FDA has not yet approved it, even though it has been used successfully in Europe for over fifteen years. Further, the use of vacuum and forceps to aid in the delivery of babies has fallen out of use in most hospitals in the Untied States because of liability concerns, which has unarguably increased the c-section rate.

The trends of what technologies are used and what technologies are not used protect maternity providers from blame in the case of bad outcomes. Why is CTG emphasized? Because it provides a visible trail of the labor and allows a provider to defend him- or herself from blame in the case of a bad outcome. Why are fetal scalp sampling and pulse oximetry not used any longer? Because they extend labors that could result in bad outcomes and liability risks to maternity providers and hospitals, as do instrumental deliveries. Why are inductions, augmentation, and epidural analgesia used rampantly? Because they allow control of labor—when it starts, how long it lasts—and a calm labor and delivery unit where women labor and give birth quickly is a unit that can be easily monitored and documented, and one where beds turn over quickly. In sum, the technologies that are used contribute to the increasing c-section rate. As physician Philip Burgin explains:

> Unless it can be a perfect vaginal delivery, I'm not interested in this one. I'm interested in doing the c-section. So, fetal monitors have to be perfect. . . . If you see any blips or anything that creates a question mark, you get delivered by c-section. The labor has to progress normally. . . . If there [are] problems with the baby coming down through the pelvis, you get a c-section. . . . We don't have them push for three or four hours anymore. We don't have patients [on whom] we use forceps or vacuums. We don't have patients [with whom] we basically go to the bitter, bitter end. . . . We need perfect results.

Women must demonstrate that they are capable of having a vaginal birth that will not put their baby in peril or their maternity providers' livelihood at risk.

PART III

The Effects of Organizational Constraints

4

The Big Kahuna

Repeat C-Sections

We are doing very few vaginal births after cesarean . . . which means that once somebody has a cesarean section, they, most of the time, get repeat cesareans, and then repeat cesareans, and it goes on and on and on.

—Physician Robert Hinson

Physician Hinson's statement is sullen, matter of fact, and true. Once a woman has a c-section, there are two ways she can give birth to a subsequent baby: repeat c-section or vaginal birth after c-section, commonly referred to as VBAC (pronounced *vee-back*). As Doctor Hinson suggests, women in the United States with a prior c-section overwhelmingly give birth by repeat c-section. In fact, one half of c-sections are performed on women with a cesarean scar.[1] VBAC has fallen significantly since its all-time high of 28.3 percent in 1996 (i.e., in 1996 28.3 percent of women who gave birth with a prior c-section had a vaginal birth) to 9.5 percent in 2004.[2] Unfortunately, the most recent national data come from 2004 because of states' use of different birth certificate forms—either the 1989 unrevised birth certificate form or the 2003 revised birth certificate form. These forms use different methods of data collection and, thus, the data collected are not all comparable, including state-level VBAC rates; hence we have no knowledge of the national VBAC rate since 2004. This is a problem highlighted by researchers at Childbirth Connection.[3] In 2010, thirty-three states used the revised form, and the VBAC rate for those states was 9.2 percent.[4] The decline in VBACs has occurred across all age, racial, and ethnic groups, and among patients with different types of health insurance.[5]

VBAC gained popularity after the 1980 U.S. National Institutes of Health (NIH) Consensus Development Conference Panel questioned the practice of routine repeat c-section and suggested situations in which VBAC should be considered.[6] The VBAC rate rose steadily from the 1980 rate of 3.4 percent until it reached the 1996 high of 28.3 percent, but it has consistently fallen since.[7] In fact, of the eighty-three postpartum women we interviewed, only two attempted a VBAC (one was successful). Although the VBAC rate continues to drop, the percentage of women who have a successful VBAC (i.e., a VBAC that ends in a vaginal birth) has not changed over time, consistently falling in the 60 to 80 percent range.[8] What this means is that 60 to 80 percent of women who attempt a VBAC have a vaginal birth.

Maternity providers—nurses, physicians, and midwives—all tell me that repeat c-sections are nearly universal among women who have had a prior c-section:

Once you have a c-section, in general, you're going to have another c-section. So the more c-sections we do now, the more repeats we're going to do in three years and [so on]. . . . We're just going to have repeats and repeats and repeats and repeats. (Nurse Eva Bunnell)

Every primary section now is one we're adding to the repeat section list. (Physician Philip Burgin)

I think once you set up a situation where the patient has a c-section, the repeat c-section is pretty standard. (Midwife Candace Whitt)

In short, VBAC is extremely rare.

A Brief History of VBAC in the United States

A bit of history might illuminate how repeat c-section has become the near-ubiquitous mode of delivery for women who have had a prior c-section. Organizations have played an important role in this change. The adage "Once a cesarean always a cesarean" is attributed to Edward Cragin's 1916 publication in the *New York Medical Journal*, although he put a name to the practice of repeat c-section, something he saw as medically necessary, so as to dissuade physicians from too quickly performing a first c-section.[9] This axiom—once a cesarean always a cesarean—remained true for decades because of the fear that in a subsequent labor the uterine scar would rupture and cause catastrophic outcomes for the woman or her baby. However, as physicians became aware that making a horizontal surgical cut in the lower uterine segment (lower transverse uterine incision) lowers the risk of rupture, as VBAC attempts were marked with success, and with the publication of the 1981 NIH Consensus Statement, more women attempted VBACs.

In 1982, shortly following the publication of the NIH Consensus Statement, ACOG issued its first VBAC guideline, and with each successive guideline issued over the next sixteen years, the restrictions on VBAC became less stringent and VBAC became more encouraged.[10] For example, the 1982 ACOG guideline indicates that VBAC is an "acceptable option" for carefully selected women giving birth in proper facilities and with appropriate staff present (i.e., an immediately available physician and anesthesiologist).[11] Then, in 1985, ACOG President Dr. L. Klein issued a press release indicating that uterine rupture is "rarely catastrophic."[12] What followed in short order were new ACOG practice guidelines in 1988, 1995, and 1998, each taking a more liberal approach to VBAC. The language on staff availability changed from being "immediately available" to being "readily available." This is an important change because immediately available was interpreted to mean that physicians and anesthesiologists must be at the hospital, whereas readily available came to be interpreted as physicians' being a phone call away. Further, whereas the 1988 guideline suggests that women should be "counseled and encouraged to attempt labor in current pregnancy," the 1994 guideline indicates "all women 'should' undergo VBAC in the absence of medical or obstetrical contraindications."[13] In short, VBAC became more encouraged

At least partly as a result of changes in guidelines and practices instigated by NIH and ACOG, the United States witnessed a period of fifteen years between 1981 and 1996 in which the VBAC rate consistently increased, reaching a high of nearly 30 percent in 1996. During this period, health insurance companies and hospitals sometimes required women to attempt a VBAC before a repeat c-section would be performed. I heard tales from physicians about this period of time. For example, physician James Montenegro tells me, "In residency we were under pressure to keep the lowest c-section rate possible. . . . At the time, I was being trained by people who were very aggressive with VBAC. . . . Every patient [with a prior c-section] had to have a VBAC."

But this tide began to turn in the late 1990s as new medical studies were published that examined the risk of uterine rupture and some accounts of devastating outcomes were highlighted in popular media.[14] Often credited with beginning the downturn in the VBAC rate is a 1996 article by Mc-Mahon and colleagues titled "Comparison of Trial of Labor with an Elective Second Cesarean Section," published in the influential *New England Journal of Medicine*, even though the article did not contain new findings about the uterine rupture rate in VBAC attempts but rather verified what had been known for several decades—a uterine rupture rate of between 0.5 and 1 percent for women with one prior lower transverse uterine scar.[15] Public attention was turned to this article, which allowed the fear of uterine rupture to become more salient in the public's mind and liability fear to become more salient in the minds of maternity providers. In our 2007 interview physician Lawrence Rascon talks about the transition away from VBAC:

> We were encouraging everybody to try to deliver vaginally after a c-section ten years ago, twelve years ago. And then as the malpractice started to go up and there were cases all over the media and in our journals of catastrophic things with the VBAC. It's going to happen. There's a one in two hundred risk of a rupture. So if you do enough of them there is going to be one, right? And as you read these things . . . you start to get afraid, and as the patients start to get a hold of these things they get afraid. . . . Because you don't get sued for doing a repeat elective cesarean section. Ever.

The interesting anomaly about the widespread attention to this article is that the reported risk of uterine rupture had not changed from the acknowledged rate established decades earlier.[16] This strange truth continues to this day. Every so often, a new article on VBAC risks is published and then receives coverage in popular news outlets. With the attention to the latest article, the public fear of uterine rupture seems to erupt again. But each of these articles still documents the same risk of uterine rupture rate that has been documented for several decades. Yet the information seems to hit the press as though uterine rupture is a newly discovered risk of VBAC attempts.

For example, in 2001 Lydon-Rochelle and colleagues' article "Risk of Uterine Rupture during Labor among Women with a Prior Cesarean Delivery," published in the *New England Journal of Medicine*, likely the most influential article on VBAC practices since the 1996 *New England Journal of*

Medicine article by McMahon and colleagues, documented a uterine rupture rate of 0.5 percent in women who attempted VBAC with spontaneous labor and 0.8 percent in women who were induced.[17] The point of this article was the authors' contention that induction of labor might increase the risk of uterine rupture, but this is not how it was portrayed in popular media, where the study was portrayed as documenting a high uterine rupture rate and the "riskiness" of VBAC.[18] Another example is a 2004 article by Landon and colleagues that documented a 0.7 percent uterine rupture risk, again a rate consistent with documented figures since the 1950s. What did not receive attention is that of the 114 uterine ruptures that occurred (out of 15,338 women who attempted VBAC), there were only 2 neonatal deaths associated with the ruptures, which is a fetal death rate due to uterine rupture of 0.013 percent.[19]

Physicians spoke with me about the irrationality of how the media spreads fear of uterine rupture:

> Even back then when everybody had to have VBAC, we would still quote a uterine rupture rate of VBAC of 1 percent or less. And we've always known that, we've always told our patients that, we've always had a consent form for that. Somehow the media, I don't know, I can't remember what year, but it was within the last eight to ten years, suddenly it just hit the press like wildfire: "Do you know that there is a 1 percent risk of uterine rupture during labor if you've had a previous c-section?" . . . There was an era eight to ten years ago where it was just constantly in the media where in a very short time suddenly it was only 10 percent of patients wanted VBAC and 90 percent were requesting repeat c-section, despite the fact that there was no change in the uterine rupture rate. It was the same number that we always quoted. Despite the fact that we have better anesthesia—at least in our hospital we have twenty-four-hour anesthesia, twenty-four-hour in-house obstetrician, an ICU, a NICU [a neo-natal intensive care unit that can care for sick babies]. As health care has gotten better, the media suddenly took away VBAC. (Physician James Montenegro)

Yet the media cannot take all the blame for curtailing VBAC. In 1999 ACOG revised its guideline on VBAC to become much more restrictive, partly as a reaction to the spate of medical articles and the public's attention to them. Though risk of uterine rupture was unchanged from when ACOG first issued VBAC guidelines in 1982, ACOG's revised VBAC guideline published in 1999 (and reaffirmed in 2004) indicates that women should be "offered" a trial of labor in contrast to earlier guidelines indicting that women should be "encouraged" to undertake a trial of labor after a previous c-section.[20] An even more dramatic change was the return to the 1982 guideline that physicians and anesthesiologists should be "immediately available" (a change from the more flexible "readily available" language in the 1988 and 1995 guidelines) in institutions that are capable of handling emergencies.[21] Specifically the bulletin indicates, "Because uterine rupture may be catastrophic, VBAC should be attempted in institutions equipped to respond to emergencies with physicians immediately available to provide emergency care."[22] Even though the 1999 guideline's recommendation of immediate availability of physicians and anesthesiologists is similar to the 1982 guideline wording, the medical–legal environment seemed to make the requirement more salient in the minds of providers than it had been in 1982.[23] Changes to ACOG practice guidelines are important because they help to establish expected practices that are often used in malpractice claims as evidence of whether an appropriate standard of care was provided.[24]

Things may be changing, although slowly. In 2010, the NIH held another Consensus Development Conference on Vaginal Birth after Cesarean Section, and in its statement the panel concludes that "given the available evidence, trial of labor is a reasonable option for many pregnant women with one prior low transverse uterine incision," and continues that there is a "paucity of high-level evidence about medical and nonmedical factors, which prevent the precise quantification of risks and benefits that might help to make an informed decision about the trial of labor compared with elective repeat cesarean delivery."[25] The panel ends with recommendations that evidence be used in decision making and that ACOG revise its recommendation for "immediately available" surgical and anesthesia personnel, given that it is not based on high-quality evidence and also that it unfairly puts uterine rupture in a different class of risk than other obstetrical emergencies.[26]

ACOG responded and issued a new Practice Bulletin in August 2010 that expands the opportunities for VBAC.[27] Among the recommendations are that women with one previous c-section and a lower transverse incision be offered a trial of labor. Further, it suggests that many women with a previous c-section should be considered candidates for a VBAC, including women with more than one previous c-section, women with suspected macrosomic babies, women with a low vertical uterine incision, women with unknown uterine scar types, and women with twin pregnancies.[28] Yet it is unlikely that VBAC attempts will significantly increase because ACOG did *not* change the resource availability language. The 2010 guidelines include the following passage: "the College recommends that TOLAC [trial of labor after cesarean] be undertaken in facilities with staff immediately available to provide emergency care."[29] When this is not possible, ACOG indicates that such a policy "cannot be used to force women to have cesarean delivery or deny care to women in labor who decline to have a repeat cesarean delivery."[30] Rather, women should be transferred to a facility that can meet the immediately available criteria for emergency care.[31] What this means, though, is that the immediately available standard has not changed. Transfer to another hospital that allows VBACs has always been a theoretical option. However, transfer is not available to all women, who may live in areas with only one hospital or be covered by health insurance that covers only certain hospitals.

Risk of VBACs, Repeat C-Sections, and First Births

This all, of course, begs the question: are VBACs riskier than repeat c-sections? There is a voluminous literature that examines this question, but there is no consensus as to what the "safest" mode of birth for a woman with a prior c-section is. This lack of consensus is traced to four intertwined facts. First, no randomized controlled trials have compared the outcomes of VBAC attempts to the outcomes of repeat c-sections, and all other research designs are prone to bias.[32] What this means is that women have not been randomly assigned to either attempt a VBAC or to have a repeat c-section. Rather, women and their maternity providers choose the mode of birth, and there is no way of knowing whether the women who attempt a VBAC and the women who have a repeat c-section are different and whether this difference may be related to outcomes.[33] Second, repeat c-sections and VBACs *both* have risks, but the risks are not directly comparable and women, depending on their age, childbearing history, and future reproductive plans, may weigh the relative importance of the risks differently.[34] Third, the risks of VBAC are increased when the VBAC attempt is not successful and an emergency c-section is performed.[35] Finally, there is no way to predict with accuracy which VBAC attempts will fail, and this lack of predictability is hampered by the lack of a randomized controlled trial.[36]

Having laid out these limitations, it is important to discuss the literature that does exist on the risks of VBAC and repeat c-section. Most of this literature focuses on the risk of uterine rupture in VBAC attempts. A c-section scar is a weakness in the uterine wall that has the potential of rupturing, or coming apart, during pregnancy or labor. What the extant literature suggests is that women who attempt a VBAC are more likely to have a uterine rupture than are women who have a repeat c-section, although all pregnant women, including women who have never given birth before, have some risk of uterine rupture.[37] This risk of uterine rupture in a VBAC attempt for a woman with a transverse (horizontal) incision in the lower part of her uterus is between 0.5 and 1 percent, while the uterine rupture risk of women who have a repeat c-section before labor begins is 0.16 percent.[38] Although the uterine rupture rates are different, the uterine rupture rate for a VBAC attempt is so low that many repeat c-sections would need to be performed to avoid even a single uterine rupture.[39]

The literature on uterine rupture risk is further complicated by the fact that most uterine scar separations that are recorded as ruptures are actually scar dehiscences, defined as a minor separation of the c-section scar with little consequence.[40] In the very rare case of a true uterine rupture—where the placenta and baby are expelled from the uterus—the baby's and the woman's lives are at risk, and an immediate c-section must be performed; however, the likelihood of a catastrophic rupture is quite slim.[41] Yet, because most studies fail to distinguish between a true scar separation and a scar dehiscence, the actual risk of catastrophic uterine rupture is hard to quantify. Here is how physician Lawrence Rascon describes this problem:

> [Uterine rupture] sounds horrible. . . . When the patients think of [uterine rupture], they think of a catastrophic rupture where the baby dies. . . . Most of these ruptures are little tears that we pick up on the monitor, and we just do a repeat section. . . . The reality is most of those little tears that happen we are in total control of them. Nothing happens to the uterus. We just sew it back up and no big deal. . . . Those would be classified as ruptures, yes, and they truly would *not* be catastrophic. The catastrophic ruptures are very rare.

As Doctor Rascon indicates, the distinction between scar dehiscence and scar rupture is important because outcomes with scar dehiscence are not catastrophic.

In fact, a baby is no more likely to die in a VBAC attempt than in a repeat c-section, yet it is this fear of a baby's dying in a VBAC attempt that drives many women to have a repeat c-section. Let me illustrate this fact with data. The combined risk of stillbirth at term and neonatal death (death during the first twenty-eight days of life) for VBAC attempts and repeat c-sections are not statistically different.[42] When only low-risk women are included in the analysis, the neonatal death rate is *higher for repeat c-sections* (1.36 per 1,000 live births) than for VBACs (1 per 1,000 live births).[43] Further, the fetal death rate due to uterine rupture in a VBAC attempt is so low (estimated to be between 2 to 4.7 per 10,000 deliveries) that *several thousand* repeat c-sections would need to be performed to prevent even one fetal death as a result of uterine rupture.[44]

There is also a new strand of medical literature arguing that comparing VBAC outcomes to repeat c-section outcomes is not appropriate because the risks are not comparable. Rather, these researchers argue that the focus to help women make decisions about how to give birth after a c-section should be on comparing the outcomes of women who attempt a VBAC to the outcomes of women who attempt a vaginal birth for the first time. When this comparison is done, it is found that neonatal and maternal morbidity rates of women attempting VBAC are similar to neonatal and maternal morbidity rates of women attempting a first vaginal birth and that fetal outcomes do not differ significantly between these groups.[45] For example, the perinatal death rate (defined as death between twenty weeks gestation and twenty-eight days of life) in VBAC births is similar to the perinatal death rate in first vaginal births.[46] In other words, a VBAC attempt is no riskier to the baby than a first-time vaginal birth.

This new way of thinking about VBAC risk highlights an interesting contradiction—we treat VBAC attempts as high risk but we do not treat women attempting vaginal birth for the first time as high risk, even though the risks are similar. Another indication of this skewed way of thinking about VBAC risk is evident when examining other unpredictable obstetrical emergencies.[47] For example, any vaginal birth has the risk of cord prolapse, where the umbilical cord drops through the vagina and is compressed by the fetus, cutting off its blood supply. The risk of fetal mortality if cord prolapse occurs is 0.1 to 0.6 percent, much higher than the fetal mortality risk in VBAC due to uterine rupture (between 0.020 and 0.047 percent), yet cord prolapse is not something maternity providers tend to focus on—hardly any mentioned this risk as a serious concern.[48]

In short, all birth has some risk—babies and women are injured and sometimes die—but the risks are slight. In fact, beyond the small risk of uterine rupture, studies suggest that fetal and maternal outcomes for women with a prior c-section attempting a vaginal delivery are similar to those who schedule a repeat c-section. The one noted exception is that maternal mortality (death), although a slight risk in any birth, is much more common in women who have a repeat c-section than in women who attempt a VBAC.[49]

This brings me to the risks of repeat c-section. Women who have a repeat c-section are much more likely to die during pregnancy or birth or within forty-two days of giving birth than are women who attempt a VBAC. Overall, women who have a repeat c-section are 3.5 times more likely to die than are women who attempt a VBAC (13.4 per 100,000 versus 3.8 per 100,000).[50] When only women at term are included in the analysis, the disparity is even more striking—women who have a repeat c-section are more than five times more likely to die from childbirth than are women who attempt VBAC (9.6 per 100,000 versus 1.9 per 100,000).[51]

As I discussed in the introductory chapter, c-sections also pose a higher risk of maternal medical complications (morbidity) than does vaginal birth and can have long-term maternal health consequences, including secondary infertility (the inability to get pregnant after already giving birth to at least one child), abnormal placentation—placenta previa (the placenta covers the cervix); placenta accreta (the placenta grows into the uterine wall and does not easily detach from the uterus); and placental abruption (the placenta ruptures before the birth)—in future pregnancies, cesarean scar ectopic pregnancy, scar adhesions, and hysterectomy, and these risks increase with each c-section.[52] Further, risks of repeat c-sections are likely higher than currently acknowledged because there is too little attention paid to the long-term maternal morbidity risks involved in repeat c-sections.[53]

Of particular concern is the link between abnormal placentation and emergency hysterectomy. The emergency hysterectomy rate is increasing, and this increase has been linked to the increasing rate of repeat c-section, likely because placenta accreta, which is becoming more and more frequent, is the most common reason that cesarean hysterectomies (hysterectomies performed immediately after a c-section) are performed.[54] These risks of abnormal placentation should not be taken lightly. In truth, in comparing morbidity risks of repeat c-sections to morbidity risks of VBACs, Makoha and colleagues in their article "Multiple Cesarean Section Morbidity," published in 2004 in *International Journal of Gynaecology and Obstetrics*, conclude, "Placenta previa and accreta, which often cause hemorrhage requiring hysterectomy, are more common and more severe causes of morbidity than uterine rupture or dehiscence."[55] In other words, the risk of placental problems caused by repeat c-sections is greater than the risk of uterine rupture in VBAC attempts.

Maternity providers commonly mentioned repeat c-section risks in their interviews. They spoke about several risks:

Abnormal placentation and hysterectomy: "After a second c-section, third, fourth, that scar, where the uterus was cut, gets thinner and thinner and thinner. And then there can be a higher chance of a placenta invading into the wall of the uterus, which you call an accreta. And if that happens, sometimes you're lucky and you can get the placenta off, but half the time you can't, and that just leads to hemorrhage, which is why it increases your chance of a cesarean hysterectomy." (Physician Rosemary Steel)

Scar tissue adhesions: "If they've had abdominal surgery of any kind—repeat c-section, myomectomy, sometimes even appendectomies, cholecystectomies—anything that would make scar tissue in the belly [that might] . . . adhere the uterus to other surrounding structures—bowel, bladder, things like that . . . they might poke a hole in the bowel; they might poke a hole in the bladder. . . . If everything's all stuck together, you have to be able to tease it away to actually get to the baby." (Nurse Eva Bunnell)

Complicated surgeries: "Repeat c-sections are like—what do I want to say—like surprise surgeries. You go, and you just have no clue about what you're going to find." (Physician Maggie Rust)

Snowballing of risk: "When someone has two, three, four, five c-sections, it gets to be very complicated with a lot of very catastrophic complications that can happen." (Physician Leticia Stites)

In other words, maternity providers are quite aware of the risk of repeat c-section. Why then is the VBAC rate so low?

Women Are Commonly Denied VBAC Opportunities

Even with all this evidence of increased risk of repeat c-section, I heard often how ACOG guideline changes caused VBAC efforts to wane. Recall that ACOG largely sets the standard of care, and with the pulling back of ACOG from encouraging VBACs, physicians and hospital administrators began to feel more of a liability threat from bad outcomes in a VBAC attempt. Some hospital administrators, perceiving that hospitals could not meet the more rigorous ACOG guidelines, forbid VBAC attempts in their institutions.[56] For example, physicians Jeffry Starling and Jacob Chism tell me:

> The American College [ACOG] changed the wording of its recommendation such that only facilities that had [immediately] available anesthesia and [operating rooms] and so forth should be doing trials of labor. [That] definitely had a kind of chilling effect on these trials of labor after cesarean deliveries. . . . That rate dropped steadily. . . . So that increased the number of repeat cesarean sections dramatically. (Physician Jeffry Starling)

> ACOG went to this immediately available standard that you have to have anesthesia and blood bank facilities immediately available, and a lot of hospitals said, "Hey, we're hearing that VBAC is more risky; we're going to have to invest all these resources in something that is only going to increase our liability." So they make an administrative decision that VBAC is not offered at their institution. . . . That's in the [corporate] suites. . . . It is a business and liability decision made at the highest levels of the organization. (Physician Jacob Chism)

Doctors Starling and Chism indicate that hospital administrators make decisions to ban VBAC attempts.

In fact, evidence suggests that after ACOG changed the VBAC guidelines in 1999, fewer hospitals offered women the opportunity to attempt a VBAC, and this change was most prominent in rural hospitals, where transfer to another hospital is often difficult due to distance.[57] A survey of California hospitals found that a majority of those covered stopped offering VBAC care because they were not able to adhere to ACOG recommendations, particularly the recommendations on staff and resources.[58] The International Cesarean Awareness Network, known as ICAN (pronounced *I can*), is conducting a multiyear project to document hospitals that ban VBAC attempts. ICAN's findings indicate that as of 2012, 30 percent of U.S. hospitals formally ban VBAC attempts.[59] As physician Jack Bianco tells me, "There [are] some hospitals, because of the fear of getting sued over ruptured uteruses with vaginal birth, won't allow [VBACs] to happen anymore."

Further, even if hospitals do not ban VBAC attempts, providers may not offer VBAC support, leading to what ICAN refers to as a "de facto" ban.[60] Although the ACOG Bulletin does not provide a definition of what it means for physicians to be "immediately available," hospital administrators commonly interpret this language to require physicians to be in the hospital, maybe even on the labor and delivery floor, when a woman attempting a VBAC is in labor.[61] That deters some physicians from allowing VBACs for their patients because it ties them to the hospital. They can no longer see patients in their offices, a more profitable activity, while a VBAC patient labors. This is particularly a problem in hospitals without hospital-employed physicians, or hospitalists, who are always present. As Jack Bianco tells me, "The hospital requirement is once a lady starts contracting . . . you bring [her] in and you have to sit there the entire time with [her]. So does this dissuade some doctors from encouraging their patients to have VBACs? You bet." Physician Christopher Froehlich has a similar perspective:

> Making rules, for example, that say if you have a woman with a previous c-section that you have to be right on the floor, not even in the cafeteria or in your office across the parking lot . . . in case there is an emergency. Well that means . . . from an economic point of view, you're tied to the hospital; you can't do anything else. . . . [They're] rules that are meant to reduce the risk for a small percentage of women, but that may make it less feasible or practical to practice the way one once did.

Physician Froehlich points out that some physicians do not support VBAC attempts because of the stringent rules imposed on the practice by hospitals.

Survey evidence suggests that physicians commonly refuse to accept VBAC patients, and hospital rules may be just one reason for this decision. ACOG's most recent survey of its members in 2012 found that 13.5 percent of responding physicians reported that they had stopped supporting VBACs (25.9 of physicians responding in 2009 reported that they had stopped supporting VBACs).[62] Another reason that physicians may not support VBACs is that their group practice may not support VBACs. Practice policies are usually established by majority vote, and if the majority of physicians in the practice do not support VBACs, typically the practice will not cover VBAC attempts. I heard from maternity providers I interviewed about practices that deny women VBAC opportunities. Physician

Christopher Froehlich tells me, "Some practices have just stopped doing VBACs. I can say that that's the case here in [suburban hospital]. . . . The busiest practice, the largest group in the community, about two or three years ago—they're just not doing any more VBACs." Similarly nurse Jane Rios says, "We only have one practice that still does [VBAC] at all. . . . A couple of practices have refused to do it because of bad outcomes or whatever in the past."

The practice effects become more problematic as practices get bigger and bigger. This has implications for many decisions because practices often set practice guidelines, including whether the practice will support VBAC patients. In addition, when malpractice suits are filed, typically every physician who has seen the woman as a patient will be named in the lawsuit. Thus, in large groups that encourage women to see as many of the physicians in the practice as possible, the risk of being sued increases because physicians see so many patients. The idea of a risk of liability when practicing in large groups is a theme evident in the way physicians thinks about VBAC:

> We know that uterine rupture will happen a finite amount of times. It's not theoretical. It happens between one in one hundred, one in two hundred births, so about one half to one percent of all births have a uterine rupture. Most of the time it is not catastrophic. But if it is, there's no second chance. You can't turn back the clock and do it a different way. . . . A busy practice . . . doing fifty to one hundred VBACs a year ultimately is going to have a problem sooner or later. They can do two hundred or three hundred without a serious problem, maybe more, but eventually the odds are it will catch up with them. (Physician Christopher Froehlich)

> So if . . . of all the VBAC attempts . . . one in one hundred or one in two hundred, somewhere in that range, are going to have catastrophes, [that is] something we are going to see every five years in our practice. . . . We can't do that and stay in practice. Remember every one of us is going to get tagged in that suit. So there's no way as a practice that we feel we can offer that to patients and still survive in this world, in this legal climate of malpractice. No way. . . . We can't accept that. (Physician Philip Burgin)

It is evident that in the minds of maternity providers a disastrous VBAC is lurking behind each successful VBAC, and they feel this risk more as practices get bigger and more women are seen by each practice.

Even hospitals and practices that continue to offer women the opportunity to attempt a VBAC have lower rates of women attempting them than in the past for a few reasons. First, although it is typical that obstetrical practices make the decision about whether they will allow women to attempt a VBAC, I have also heard of practices in which some of the physicians in the practice will support a woman's attempting a VBAC and some will not. For example, if in a practice of five physicians, two physicians will support VBAC attempts and three will not, a woman will be allowed the opportunity to attempt a VBAC only if one of the two supportive physicians is on call when she comes into the hospital in labor. If one of the other three is on call, she will have a repeat c-section. Nurse April Coleman mentions this: "There's another group that has five physicians in it, and one will do it [VBAC]. So any patient in that group that would want to attempt [a VBAC] would have to attempt it with that physician." Similarly, physician Lois Timberlake warns patients about this practice:

> I had a patient come to me yesterday who had two previous c-sections, wanted a VBAC, and was saying, "If I come to your practice, will I be able to have a VBAC?" and I had to be very honest with her and say, "You know, we're in a big group, and we practice obstetrics as a group," that I certainly could not guarantee that if she came in in labor that every one of my partners would be willing to allow labor.

Thus, finding a supportive physician may not be enough. A woman who wants to attempt a VBAC must make sure that every physician in the practice is supportive of VBAC.

Second, the ACOG guidelines also affect the management of women attempting a VBAC. The 1999 ACOG bulletin requires strict management of women attempting a VBAC such that some physicians will not induce or augment labor or allow women to be monitored intermittently. Induction and augmentation are much debated in the literature and there is no consensus as to whether they increase the risk of uterine rupture or whether different induction agents increase the rupture rate, but physicians are still hesitant to manage women in this way because the ACOG Bulletin notes this ambiguity and does not strongly support these practices.[63] Women are carefully watched for signs of trouble. This vigilance is not consistent with empirical evidence on risk of uterine rupture or with how first-time mothers are managed, even though they have similar risks of perinatal death. ACOG has defined VBAC as "different" and "high risk." Once this social definition is applied, as we see from the declining VBAC rate, it has real consequences.

Third, obstetrical practices that support VBAC may allow only women who meet stringent criteria to attempt a VBAC. Nurse Genevieve Caesar tells me, "We have some groups that don't do them at all and some that . . . have stringent criteria." These criteria include:

Only women with one previous c-section: "I'm still willing to do VBACs. . . . We used to allow them . . . if you had two sections; now it only has to be one. Otherwise you're not eligible." (Physician Janice Obrien)

Only women who come into the hospital by their due dates in spontaneous labor: "They all have different comfort levels. So some of them will say, 'Well, if you come in, in good, spontaneous labor all on your own before your due date, you can go ahead and try VBAC.'" (Nurse Eva Bunnell)

Only women who have had a previous vaginal birth (a "proven pelvis"): "If someone's had a previous vaginal delivery and then a c-section, I think [my partners] would all be willing to do it." (Physician Lois Timber-lake)

Although women with one prior c-section who go into spontaneous labor and who have had a previous vaginal birth may be more likely to have a successful VBAC, there is no empirical model that successfully *predicts* which women will be successful.[64]

Survey evidence documents that indeed many women are denied VBAC opportunities. Recall that ICAN has documented that 30 percent of U.S. hospitals formally ban VBAC and others have "de facto" bans. When examining women's actual experiences, the LTMII survey indicates that 45 percent of women giving birth after a previous c-section were interested in VBAC but that a majority of those women (57 percent) were denied the opportunity because of an unwilling provider (45 percent) and/or an un-willing hospital (23 percent).[65] There are also many documented accounts of women's being forced to have a repeat c-section because they could not find a provider or a hospital that would allow VBAC.[66]

In our sample of women, sixteen women had a previous c-section, and of those women ten (62.5 percent) were denied a VBAC opportu-nity. Eight (50 percent) had more than one previous c-section and one (6 percent) was pregnant with twins, both situations in which many maternity providers will not offer women the opportunity to have a VBAC, and this was the case for all of these women—none were offered a VBAC opportunity. Three (19 percent) chose a repeat c-section, two (13 percent) chose a VBAC attempt (one was successful), and one (6 percent) had a repeat c-section and was not offered the choice to have a VBAC (one woman [6 percent] had a repeat c-section but was not clear whether she had a VBAC opportunity). Thirty-three-year-old Heidi tells us, "I wasn't even given the opportunity [for a VBAC], because my cervix never opens past a certain amount. . . . I never really put thought into it because it was never an option." Ella, a thirty-year-old woman, relays a similar story when she says, "I wasn't given an option [to have a VBAC]. My doctor told me 'We're going to do a repeat because we did it with the last one.'" It is likely that these tales of women not being offered a VBAC opportunity are quite common.

The Real Risk

Although I am quite sympathetic to the risk providers feel by attending VBAC attempts, it is also important to point out important nuances in how they are assessing risk. First, the doctor's risk of overseeing a VBAC in which a uterine rupture occurs is not the same as a woman's risk that she will have a uterine rupture in a VBAC attempt. In other words, a physician experiences a different "lifetime" risk of uterine rupture over his or her career than does a woman in her one-time risk of having a uterine rupture in a VBAC attempt.

When physicians oversee a number of successful VBACs, because they are assessing risk based on their own risk, they may worry that a bad outcome is just around the corner. Using this type of logic to assess *a woman's risk* of uterine rupture is an error because the chance of independent events is not linked with preceding chances of the same event. For example, gamblers who play games of luck (like a slot machine) and believe that they will win the next game because they have lost three games in a row exhibit this fallacy of logic. The chance of winning a game is independent of the whether the previous game was won or lost. If the chance of winning a slot machine is one in one hundred, that chance of winning remains the same, regardless of how many times the individual has already won or lost. This fallacy also clouds the logic of physicians who believe that if they have overseen several successful VBAC patients in a row, a uterine rupture must be around the next corner. This is not how statistical probability works. *Each woman attempting a VBAC has a uterine rupture risk of between 0.5 and 1 percent, regardless of how many successful VBACs that precede her* with a certain provider, in a certain hospital, in a certain state, and so forth. Her risk is independent.

It is the case that a physician should expect that in every two hundred VBAC attempts a uterine rupture would happen. But, again, this risk is for the physician, not the woman. What this means is that if a physician oversees thousands of VBACs over a career, he or she will likely see a few uterine ruptures, more than a physician who oversees less than one hundred VBAC attempts. This is different from the chances a women will experience a uterine rupture in her VBAC attempt, which is always a 0.5 to 1 percent risk. It is clear, then, that the way doctors are assessing risk elevates self-interest over the mother's interests.

Second, providers' understanding of risk suggests that "bad outcomes" happen in one out of every one hundred or two hundred births. But remember that the uterine rupture statistic includes scar dehiscences, which are minor separations of the uterine scar with little consequence. In other words, the providers have the uterine rupture rate correct (0.5–1 percent), but most uterine ruptures are *not catastrophic*. Babies are unlikely to die due to uterine rupture in a VBAC attempt: the rate is 2 to 4.7 per 10,000 deliveries. Further, recall that the risk of a baby's dying is not higher in a VBAC birth than in a repeat c-section, and when only low-risk women are examined, repeat c-sections actually have a slightly higher neonatal mortality rate than do VBAC births.[67] It is also the case that maternal morbidity and neonatal morbidity and mortality rates are the same for women attempting VBAC and for women giving birth vaginally for the first time.[68] In short, VBAC births do not have a one in one hundred or two hundred risk of a *catastrophic outcome*.

Finally, the way providers are assessing risk is also prone to selective perception—sometimes called confirmation bias—which is when individuals pay attention most to cases that support their point of view.[69] This would happen, for example, if a person were to favor strict gun control and, thus, notice cases in which guns are obtained legally and used violently. They would, on the other hand, ignore when legally purchased guns were used safely and nonviolently. In the case of VBAC attempts, maternity providers may be prone to this bias and, thus, remember most those few VBAC attempts that ended badly, while ignoring the many more cases of successful VBAC attempts.

The Role of Organizations

Organizations are clearly guiding the decline of VBACs, from ACOG to hospitals to medical practices. In particular the role of ACOG guidelines in restricting VBAC opportunities is concerning for a few reasons. First, there is a lack of consistency in national guidelines on vaginal birth after c-section, an indication that there is no international consensus on best practices concerning VBAC.[70] In other words, women's choices are being constrained when there is not widespread agreement on how best to handle VBACs. Second, there is a lack of high-quality evidence that having surgical and anesthesia staff immediately available makes surgery quicker and outcomes better.[71] This guideline is based on Level C evidence—consensus and expert opinion—the weakest form of evidence that exists in medical research. Level C evidence is equivalent to what maternity providers "think" is best and is not based on scientific evidence of improved outcomes. Level A evidence is the best—good and consistent scientific evidence—followed by Level B evidence—limited or inconsistent scientific evidence. The difference between "readily available" and "immediately available" is important because "immediately available" came to be defined as anesthesiologists, obstetricians, and operating rooms being available during the entire labor of a VBAC patient. Many hospital administrators and maternity providers decided they couldn't meet this strict guideline and banned or refused to support VBAC attempts.[72]

In short, ACOG guidelines have driven the VBAC rates, and these guidelines are tied to liability threats. In 2001 Stanley Zinberg, then vice president of Practice Activities of ACOG, published an article in *Obstetrics and Gynecology* in which he defended the conservative changes in the 1999 Practice Bulletin. In his defense of the "immediately available" of personnel and resources requirement, he suggested that it is necessary to deal with the liability threat: "Based on reports from members of ACOG, uterine rupture almost always results in legal action, no matter what the clinical outcome and no matter how excellent the clinical care. Defendant physicians are in a better position from a liability perspective if they were present at the time of the complications."[73] What this suggests is that ACOG officials know that the "immediately available" requirement means that fewer women will have access to VBAC. However, they acknowledge that they must have this requirement, not to improve maternal or fetal outcomes but rather so that maternity providers are able to better defend themselves against a malpractice liability claim. For maternity providers, it is legally safer to be present when a bad outcome happens. Thus at least part of the reason for this "readily available" requirement is to deal with perceived liability threats. This is how maternity providers talk about liability and VBAC:

> If you look at doing vaginal deliveries after having a cesarean section, we used to do that routinely. It used to be preferred. We used to encourage it. Now, most doctors don't even accept patients who want to have a vaginal birth after a cesarean. They just will go right to a repeat cesarean section. So, I mean that's changed over the past ten years and that's surely liability driven. That has nothing to do with reality. (Physician Leticia Stites)

> We don't do vaginal deliveries after c-section. If you've had one c-section, you have all c-sections. . . . Patients come to us and say they want a VBAC. We say, "No. Go somewhere else, if you can find somebody else." There are not too many that do that anymore because it is so dangerous. And every single [person who] has a catastrophe with a VBAC sues their doctors. Every single one. Despite what they sign, what they know. (Physician Philip Burgin)

> We did the VBACs for a while, and now they won't even consider them. Too risky. And my question to [physicians] is, "Do you think it's medically risky or do you think it's legally risky?" And they say, "Well, there is of course the statistical medical risk but legally, there is no room. If you let a woman VBAC who then has trouble [you will be asked], "Why didn't you section her?" There's no legal recourse. There's no defense." (Nurse Amanda Barnett)

Physicians have learned—from hospitals, from the media, from ACOG—that VBACs are risky and that they should avoid them, an example of how control structures guide decisions even though the structures may not be apparent. Providers anticipate negative consequences if they support VBACs and there is a bad outcome. This problem is simply not there with repeat c-sections. It is easy to see the allure then for maternity providers of repeat c-sections.

Other organizations, besides ACOG, hospitals, practices, and the media, also have a hand in this trend. What may not be recognized is that often the reason hospitals and practices do not offer women VBAC opportunities is because their malpractice insurers have said they will not cover negative birth outcomes associated with a VBAC attempt.[74] Thus malprac-tice insurers are also setting policies that restrict women's access to VBAC. I heard this from a number of maternity providers:

I don't think it's as much the willingness of the provider as the willingness of the provider's malpractice insurance carrier. . . . That's just the plain, honest truth about it. (Nurse Diana Ainsworth)

Now for the [malpractice] insurance companies who are covering doc-tors, they want to see the VBAC rate as zero because VBACs for insurance companies are huge losers because they are big-ticket items. (Physician Joe Haley)

The hospitals won't even let me do VBACs. I used to do them all the time. I did them for twenty years, actually. But I'm no longer allowed to do them. . . . The [malpractice] insurance company dictates to the hospital. They say if we're paying, if he has a problem we're not going to cover it. . . . They can say it would be a non-covered event. (Physician Christopher Freulich, employed by a hospital)

Thus malpractice insurers clearly have a hand in the VBAC decline as well.

Reinsurance companies are also organizations that may refuse insurance coverage for groups that support VBAC. This is how reinsurance works: a primary insurance company, such as a malpractice insurer, buys a policy that insures the company against large claims—for example, claims over $2 million. In other words, reinsurers offer insurance policies to malprac-tice insurance companies. The primary insurer reduces revenues by buying such a policy, but buying a reinsurance policy limits its liabilities in large claims and decreases the risk of insolvency.[75] It is common for malpractice insurance companies to buy reinsurance because malpractice claims are not filed often, but when they are they are filed for large amounts, making actuarial predictions difficult.[76] This tendency for malpractice insurers to buy reinsurance policies is indicative of the uncertainty they face, and it is also a view into how multiple layers of organizations may affect health care delivery. What that means is that there are two levels of insurers setting policies—the malpractice insurance company and the reinsurance com-pany. Physician Andrew Robinette explains the role of reinsurers:

In my group we decided we needed to do something about [the liability crisis]. That's why we formed our own insurance company. So I have the opportunity to talk to a certain group of people who are just pure risk managers [and] . . . reinsurers. These are people like Lloyd's of London and Transatlantic Reinsurance and Hanover and all these places all over the world. And for them the higher the c-section rate is, the better. The lower the VBAC rate is, [the better]. The first question they always ask me [is], "You guys don't do VBACs do you?" . . . From a risk point of view, all you need is a few bad cases, and it costs a lot of money, and they can lose their shirts on it. These people are investing in insurance. (Physician Andrew Robinette)

In essence, then, reinsurance companies—companies that most women know nothing about—restrict women's birth options.

Conclusion

In sum, there are a variety of levels at which women are denied the opportunity to attempt a VBAC—it can be denied by physicians, practices, hospitals, malpractice insurers, or reinsurers. What this means is that there are many, many women in this country who do not have the opportunity to attempt a VBAC even though it is a perfectly prudent and reasonable choice to do so, particularly for women who want to have more children.

The jury is still out on whether the 2010 ACOG guidelines will significantly change the VBAC rate. Many are not optimistic that change will happen with the immediately available recommendation still in place.[77] In fact, it is quite disturbing to find ACOG officials justifying their refusal to change the language in the guideline, ignoring the NIH recommendation, because of liability threats. As reported by Bridget M. Kuehn, Hal C. Lawrence, vice president of Practice Activities for ACOG, stated at the NIH conference, "Unless there are some liability changes, backing off the 'immediately available' position is very problematic."[78] The question must be, "Problematic for whom?"

I am also pessimistic that the new NIH report and ACOG's revised statement will make much of a difference in the VBAC rate. Women may still have great difficulty finding maternity providers, practices, and hospitals that allow VBAC attempts. VBAC is a practice that must be addressed much more strongly than ACOG addressed it in the organization's 2010 practice guidelines. Because the practice has withered, it will not so easily grow back. For example, survey evidence indicates that younger maternity providers are less likely to offer VBAC, indicating that a concerted effort must be made to increase training opportunities for young physicians to attend VBACs and see their success.[79]

In short organizations have defined repeat c-sections as a panacea for liability threat. The authoritative control may be more apparent for repeat c-sections than for primary c-sections, but both are guided by what Carl J. Friedrich calls "the rule of anticipated reaction."[80] In order to avoid negative consequences, maternity providers have learned from organizations that VBAC births are to be avoided.

5

Women's Lack of Choice in Labor and Birth

[There is] a shift in society where people have become sort of their own professionals. And people now have a lot more input [in decisions about their medical care], whether they understand something or not, about what happens to them. . . . I would say that the changes in society probably happened throughout medicine—not just in obstetrics—but probably in all aspects of medicine. If you've gone to the doctor, I'm sure you have been given more choices in terms of your therapeutic options than, let's say, your grandmother or even your mother.
—Physician Allen Homan

Physician Homan is correct about this shift in society, which has been pointed out by medical sociologists as a move toward a consumer relationship between physicians and patients, with patients having more autonomy to make health care choices.[1] This idea of choice in birth is rampant in the stories we commonly hear about reproduction. Women are told they can choose abstinence, birth control, abortion, in vitro fertilization, c-sections, and the list goes on and on. Choice is consistent with the American focus on neoliberal individualism, yet scholars of reproduction have pulled apart this rhetoric of choice to suggest that choice is not always available to women, and that when it is available it may not be available to all women.[2] Take for example abortion, which states like South Dakota are close to outlawing. Women with the necessary financial resources may have the ability to cross the state border and obtain an abortion in Minnesota, but that choice may not be available to women with low incomes. These women do not have a choice to have a legal abortion. Another example is that women who seek abortions in Louisiana and Texas must have an ultrasound before the abortion, and the abortion providers are required to both show and describe the ultrasound image to the women.[3] Women do not have the choice to refuse the ultrasound. Yet another example is that many women cannot choose in vitro fertilization, a common way that infertile heterosexual couples and gay and lesbian couples conceive biological children, because not all states mandate that health insurance companies pay for this costly procedure, and, even if they do, not all women have health insurance. This framework of being critical about the reproductive choices women have is tied to the reproductive justice movement, perhaps most strongly promoted by the Atlanta-based organization SisterSong Women of Color Reproductive Justice Collective.[4] This movement asserts that reproductive justice requires economic and social justice. Without justice on these levels, choice becomes impossible, because choice is simply not present for many women.

In this chapter I explore the ways in which women lack choice in modern maternity care and how this lack of choice contributes to the c-section epidemic because women cannot avoid unnecessary c-sections and interventions that lead to c-sections. For example, as I demonstrated earlier, women are told they must have a c-section because of CTG tracings that are wrong 99.8 percent of the time. Women are told they must be induced or have a c-section because their babies are "too big" when there is no accurate way to predict fetal weight. Women are told they must have a c-section because they have been pushing "too long" even though a vaginal birth may still be possible. And women cannot find maternity providers and hospitals that will allow them to attempt a VBAC, a vaginal twin birth, or a vaginal breech birth. In short, women are not given a choice about how their babies will be born. I explore the concept of "choice" broadly construed, as related to labor and birth, and show how the concept is fraught with contradictions.[5] It is not just maternity providers who feel they lack choices, as I have discussed most in the book. Those at the heart of the matter, pregnant women, also lack choice in modern maternity care.

Women "Choose" Repeat C-Sections?

An example of the lack of choice that women face is with VBAC. VBAC was a prominent theme in the interviews. Given the organizational constraints women face in finding providers, practices, and hospitals that will support VBAC attempts, it was surprising to find in my interviews that many maternity providers believe women "choose" to have a repeat c-section rather than attempt a VBAC. Here are some examples of ways that physicians talk about repeat c-sections that puts the blame squarely on the shoulders of women, without complicating the issue of how the decision might have been made:

I definitely see one of the reasons why the [c-section] rate is higher is because of repeat c-sections. So, you know, a lot of women choose to do a repeat c-section for different reasons. (Physician Rosemary Steel)

I just see [the c-section rate] going higher and higher because, again, as you're doing more sections for things that we used to deliver vaginally, those are all repeat sections [and] because you're not going to change the woman's mind about repeat section, I don't think. (Physician Lawrence Rascon)

Some women may choose a repeat c-section, but there is no evidence that 91 percent choose a repeat c-section over a VBAC attempt. Survey evidence documents that indeed many women are denied VBAC opportunities. Recall ICAN has documented that 30 percent of U.S. hospitals formally ban VBAC and that others have "de facto" bans. Further, the LT-MII survey indicates that 45 percent of women giving birth after a previous c-section were interested in VBAC but more than half of them (57 percent) were denied the opportunity.[6] In my sample, sixteen women had a previous c-section and ten (62.5 percent) were denied the opportunity to attempt a vaginal birth. There are also many documented accounts of women being forced to have a repeat c-section because they could not find a provider or a hospital that would allow VBAC.[7]

Another way that women's choices are constrained about whether to attempt a VBAC or schedule a repeat c-section is the way information is presented to them. An important study by Sarah N. Bernstein, Shira Matalon-Grazi, and Barak M. Rosenn was published in 2012 in *American Journal of Obstetrics and Gynecology* examining how women makes choices about having a VBAC or repeat c-section.[8] The authors concluded that most women who are candidates for a VBAC know little about the risks and benefits associated with VBAC and repeat c-section and rather are heavily swayed by their providers' preferences.[9] When patients believed their doctors preferred them to deliver by repeat c-section, they chose this option 86 percent of the time.[10] (On the other hand, when patients believed their doctors preferred VBAC, they chose that option 78 percent of the time.[11] Such a finding calls into question whether these women are adequately informed enough about their options to consider the decisions they make "choices." This could happen in several ways. For example, in the interviews of postpartum women, women talked of how repeat c-section was portrayed to them as less risky than a VBAC attempt:

[My physician] didn't tell me, "This is what you should do." . . . She gave me . . . percentages of babies who don't make it, of mothers who don't make it. . . . Then she explained to me, too, that if I try to labor and then I end up with a c-section anyway, now I've increased my risks even more because now I've thinned things out by trying to push in labor. . . . When I left the office that day, I knew [repeat c-section] was what I wanted to do. (Kathy)

From Kathy's account, the risk of VBAC was explained perhaps to the exclusion of risk of repeat c-section. This is indicative of another way that risk comes into play with VBAC: consent forms have become very detailed and typically list the risks of VBAC, but often do not cover as extensively the risks of repeat c-section. These consent forms are commonly talked about by maternity providers as "scary," and some clinicians suggest that "there is often an unspoken undercurrent that a repeat cesarean delivery is essentially without risk."[12]

I heard from many maternity providers that the VBAC informed consent forms steer women to repeat c-sections, particularly in the way providers present these forms. Communication of risks is essential, and if providers are concerned about the legal risks of VBAC attempts it seems fair to question how they are presenting to women the risks of VBAC attempts compared to the risks of repeat c-sections. Literature suggests that women are heavily swayed by such presentations, and it is apparent that the presentation is often intended to encourage women to acquiesce to the providers' delivery preference, often a repeat c-section.[13] Further, interview evidence suggests that maternity providers often use evidence to justify their views rather than as a tool in objective decision making.[14] This type of evidence usage and presentation of risk was commonly discussed in interviews. Midwife Joyce Linville laments:

People [should] understand, at least in the case of vaginal birth after cesarean, that it's not risk versus no risk. It's different kinds of risk and what kinds of risk are you willing to tolerate as a patient? But it's not being presented that way. I think most people have the idea that a c-section is clean; it's safe; it's without risk; and it's always the right thing to do.

Similarly, physician Tony Oday says, "Everybody has a huge concern with VBAC, . . . even [though] the risks may be small, because of the issue of liability. . . . We're counseling patients differently today than we were before all that new information came out, even though [risk] really wasn't that different."

Part of the reason an uneven presentation may occur is that physicians are fearful of liability and are not confident that consent forms will be enforced in the case of a bad outcome. Physician Jack Bianco describes this sentiment:

> The patient can say, "I didn't understand it. If I really knew I could die if my uterus ruptured, I wouldn't have done this." Or the person's estate says they didn't really know. What if the husband disagrees with the wife and didn't want her to do it; she signs; it's her body; she dies. The husband can sue me for having done something that he didn't think his wife understood. It's up to the jury to decide. So consents are better than no consents, and good consents are better than bad consents. And you definitely do have people sign for consent for vaginal birth after cesarean. Does it scare some people away? You betcha it does. But guess what? I did not ask for it to be so stringent, and so rigid, and so scary to people. Society asked for it to be that way. . . . It's a very challenging situation.

It is important to understand the very real threat providers feel from VBAC. They feel there will necessarily be some bad outcomes, as there is always a risk in birth, but in the case of VBAC they feel the risk is more apparent and that they will be held accountable regardless of whether a consent form was signed. In such a situation, it is easy to see how providers may steer women to repeat c-section.

When women are asked after a repeat c-section about the birth, evidence suggests that many would have chosen VBAC if they had been given the opportunity.[15] Other survey evidence suggests that women who have a repeat c-section would prefer to have a vaginal delivery for their next birth, and that over 40 percent of women express a preference for a vaginal birth for their next birth within six months of their c-section.[16] In other words, the idea that women "choose" c-sections is a myth, and suggesting so is a failure to adequately acknowledge the role of organizations in taking away women's options for VBAC.

Women "Choose" C-Sections Because They're Safer?

It's not just repeat c-sections that women are believed to choose. It is also common for maternity providers to emphasize that c-sections are safer than vaginal births and to suggest that women choose to have c-sections for this reason. Recall from the introduction that there is a rather common belief, especially among maternity providers, that women choose to have non-medically indicated c-sections (the "too posh to push" argument), even though there is no empirical evidence that women commonly choose c-sections without medical indications. Extending this idea of women's choosing to schedule non-medically indicated c-sections to women's making the choice during labor to have a c-section, it must be questioned just exactly how c-sections are being portrayed to women. What I found in my interviews of maternity providers is that c-sections are talked about as "safe" and a way to prevent bad outcomes in birth. This presentation, of course, stands in stark contrast to empirical evidence of increased fetal and maternal mortality and morbidity for c-sections.[17] Thus, if c-sections are portrayed to women as safe and a woman decides during labor to have a c-section, is that really a "choice"? This presentation of c-sections as "safe" was common in my interviews. For example, physician Eric Kraemer sees c-sections as safe:

As technology got better and [a] cesarean [section] got to be a much safer and a much more routine operation, I think it no longer was weighing a bad baby versus a bad mother outcome. Now it looked like, gee, we could do a c-section for most people with minimum of stress and strain and, yes, . . . a longer time recuperating, but at least we know in the long run [that] this mother's going to do fine, and we have less worry about the baby . . . struggling through twenty-four hours of difficult labor and maybe having a damaged baby delivered.

C-sections have been socially constructed as a way to prevent risk to the baby, even though this idea is not supported by empirical data. It is a myth, but a myth with real consequences. As long as c-sections are perceived as preventing bad outcomes and of being safe to women and babies, even safer than vaginal birth, c-sections become acceptable. Physician Joe Haley also talks about c-sections as being safe and a way to prevent bad outcomes:

The reality is that cesarean section in a hospital like [City] Hospital, and most modern hospitals, is a very, very low-risk operation. And if you're going to really prevent a life long disability for a baby, then I think the trade off is for many situations worth it to do a cesarean section because the recovery . . . [a] very high percentage of the time is very good. It's definitely more painful; it definitely causes some short-term disability that's longer than a vaginal delivery; but there [are] very, very few major catastrophes with a cesarean section just because regional anesthesia is used so often. . . . Even if we had actually no liability, I think we would have a creep up in the cesarean section rate because people are . . . not going to be happy with even a small chance of a problem with the forceps delivery, a problem with a vacuum delivery, or that really small chance of the baby not getting enough oxygen during labor.

Notice how Doctor Haley focuses here on how patients aren't happy with the risks of forceps or vacuum extraction or the potential that a baby's not getting enough oxygen in labor (he's referring here to a non-reassuring CTG strip). His words make it appear that women choose c-sections for these reasons. Yet one could only consider this a choice if the risks of c-section are presented fairly and not minimized. Thus, if women decide on c-sections without hearing such a presentation of risk, can that really be considered a choice?

Another interesting aspect of this excerpt is Doctor Haley's focus on the safety of c-sections for women, particularly because of the use of regional anesthesia—an epidural or a spinal. General anesthesia is used in some c-sections, for example, if the surgery must be done quickly or if a woman who has regional anesthesia begins to feel pain during the surgery. In our sample of eighty-three woman, thirty-one had c-sections and three of those women (or 9.6 percent of women who had c-sections) had general anesthesia, slightly higher than the 7 percent of women in the LTMII survey who reported being put under general anesthesia for c-sections.[18] In other words, the use of general anesthesia in c-sections *does* happen, and even with regional anesthesia, c-sections are not as safe for women and babies as is vaginal birth.

"Choosing" C-Sections: It's All about the Baby

Almost all physicians I interviewed held the belief that a c-section is safer for the baby than is a vaginal birth. One maternity provider even told me that "babies love being born by cesarean section." Although as recently as 2006 the U.S. National Institutes of Health State-of-the-Science Conference on Maternal Request for Cesarean Sections concluded that there is no evidence that suggests a clear answer to whether a planned vaginal or planned c-section birth is safer for babies and women, empirical evidence now clearly challenges that statement—even for babies. Recall from the introduction of the book that José Villar and colleagues found that elective c-sections are associated with higher rates of maternal morbidity and mortality and fetal death than are planned vaginal births.[19] Further, Marian MacDorman and colleagues compared neonatal mortality rates in planned vaginal births and planned c-sections in the United States and found a higher neonatal death rate in planned c-sections than in planned vaginal births, by a rate of 1.69–2.4 times.[20]

Interestingly, because of the common belief that c-sections are safer for babies than are vaginal births, physicians were quick to emphasize the safety of c-sections even though they are aware that c-sections have the potential to harm women, although as discussed above, the risk of c-sections to women is still deemphasized. In other words, they emphasize the health of the baby over the health of the mother. How risk to women and risk to babies are weighed is not decided by promoting the health of the baby in isolation. Rather, I find that maternity providers' calculus of risk closely relates to their perceived liability risk. In a nutshell, part of the reason maternity providers emphasize the health of the baby over the health of the woman is that they perceive, with some accuracy, that they will more likely be sued for a poor fetal outcome than for a poor maternal outcome.[21] Maternity providers display such a calculus in a number of ways. Several maternity providers—midwives and physicians—discussed how liability risk permeates the weighing of damage to the baby versus damage to the woman. Some are reflexive and critical about this calculus:

> It seems like we're all so obsessed with a healthy baby, a perfect birth, preventing birth trauma and that type of thing. . . . It is almost like at the expense of the women, because you know that either they're not going to have a better birth experience—there is more risk with a c-section . . . higher risk of having a hysterectomy or bleeding during surgery and things like that. And maybe that is something that is not taken into consideration. . . . [Physicians are] more about having that perfect birth and a healthy baby because I think that is where liability typically falls. If things don't go well, if the birth is difficult, if there is anything wrong with that baby, so many people come back later and attach it to the birth. (Midwife Ada Medlin)

Physicians have integrated this way of calculating risk, even in very specific ways, into how they think about c-sections and what an "acceptable" c-section rate is. Physician Jeffrey Starling eloquently suggests how this may occur:

You have to ask a question, what is an acceptable rate of cesarean delivery to prevent one fetal intrauterine death or one case of cerebral palsy? And if the majority of practitioners feel that fetal distress unrelenting will either lead to death or cerebral palsy . . . and they'll get a $40 million suit for sitting on that and they would feel horrible personally at having a dead baby or a brain-damaged baby—then the answer may well be not only is 10:1 acceptable, 100:1 would be acceptable, maybe even 1,000:1 would be acceptable. So what I think we need to begin to put into the calculus as well is, "OK, but if a woman wants to have more than two kids, what about the risk of placenta previa, the risk of her hemorrhaging to death, or the risk of her losing her uterus and needing multiple [blood] transfusions if she has her third or fourth or fifth cesarean delivery . . . or the risk of catastrophic rupture?" and so forth.

Starling highlights how the calculation of risk often leaves out risk to the health of the woman. Providers readily talk about how risk calculus of c-sections is influenced by perceptions of liability risk:

If you have a complication with a c-section, as long as a woman doesn't die, almost any complication they suffer to give birth to this baby they are going to tolerate. And they're going to say, "Well, this is what we had to do to get this baby out." So they had pulmonary embolism, they had an infection, they had a wound break open, they had a bladder laceration that had to be fixed. These are not happy things, but the women are willing to suffer this for their babies, like they will do . . . tons of things for their babies. Ask any mother who cares about [her] baby, "Would you suffer something to make sure this baby [is] healthy?" Of course, you would do it. So they're not going to sue for those things. Again, a mother dying is a big problem. But all or most of the complications of c-sections, people aren't going to sue for. But a bad baby they're going to sue for. (Physician Philip Burgin)

The reality is [that] cesarean section is really, really safe, overall. It is a major operation—it definitely is risky surgery—infection, bleeding, injury to organs next to the uterus when you're doing a cesarean section—but every doctor knows that almost all things that can go wrong at a cesarean section are small-ticket items compared to being accused of not doing a cesarean section that could have prevented this baby's brain damage. (Physician Joe Haley)

There is a big concern if you have a surgical complication [to the mother] because of cesarean. . . . You get sued [but] it still is unlikely to be the same sort of suit as a bad baby. So a surgical complication may be worth thousands of dollars or even hundreds of thousands of dollars, but not millions of dollars, so that's a big difference in people's mind-sets. (Physician Maggie Rust)

In short, maternity providers' calculation of risk is heavily influenced by their understanding that liability risk is much higher for a damaged baby than for a damaged woman and that by performing a c-section they have done everything they could to assure the baby's health. Yet the empirical data suggest that c-sections are more dangerous to women and babies. Do women know this?

Women's Information on Labor and Birth

As I argued in the last chapter, women do not have good information about the risks of repeat c-section and VBAC. I extend that argument here to suggest more generally that few women have a good understanding of labor and birth or the interventions used in labor and birth, and this complicates their ability to make choices in labor and birth. The most accurate and reliable data on the information women have about childbirth come from the LTMII survey.[22] Only one quarter of women who completed the survey took childbirth classes, and of these women, 87 percent took the classes at a hospital or at a maternity provider's office.[23] Independent childbirth classes are more rare. Childbirth classes in hospitals have been demonstrated to legitimize the role of technology and interventions in assuring a safe birth, whereas independent childbirth classes are shown to give a more balanced view of birth.[24] This truth is born out in the LTMII survey, which found that childbirth classes led women to have greater trust in hospitals (60 percent) and have less fear of interventions (54 percent).[25] Women we interviewed talked about the hospital childbirth classes they took as informative but scary. For example, Gina tells us about the hospital-based childbirth class she took. She talks about how she learned what could go wrong during labor and birth:

GINA: I took a childbirth preparation class from [City] Hospital. . . . They had some material, which was helpful.

INTERVIEWER: What did they go over in that class?

GINA: That class was . . . actually more about what you can expect. It wasn't like a Lamaze class or breathing class. It was really more about preparation for childbirth, which I appreciated.

HUSBAND: I called it the scare-tactics class.

INTERVIEWER: The scare-tactics class?

GINA: Yeah. Because it was truly—here is what you should expect during labor. It was more the technical, physical aspects of labor. Things like there's good reason why you may have to have a c-section. If you do, here are the reasons why and here is what you might expect. Things like that. Just real honest to goodness—these are the things that could happen.

Gina's experience in a hospital-based childbirth education class is consistent with literature that suggests these classes tend to normalize interventions and c-sections rather than intervention-free vaginal birth.[26]

Whereas few women who completed the LTMII survey took childbirth classes, a majority of women watched television shows depicting birth (68 percent) and used the Internet at some point in pregnancy to seek out information on pregnancy and birth (76 percent).[27] Research shows that the majority of women who use the Internet during pregnancy do so to find information to make decisions about their pregnancies.[28] Further, a 2012 study in *Gender and Society* by Felicia Wu Song and colleagues found that women used information from the Internet on pregnancy and birth that reinforced the dominant medical model of birth and, importantly, that they continued to rely on their doctors in decision making.[29] Further, information presented on television and available on the Internet varies starkly in reliability, and media representations are particularly biased presentations of labor and birth. Analyses of reality television programs about birth have found that labor and birth are displayed as fraught with danger, and that these programs portray doctors using technology to save babies from the perils of birth.[30] Bad outcomes are seldom shown, and birth is overwhelmingly medicalized, showing women who have received epidurals and are pushing on their backs. Importantly, c-sections are overrepresented.[31] Yet reality television shows are a major source of information for birthing women.[32] Charlene, a woman we interviewed, suggests that the videos shown in her childbirth education class were outdated and did not show what birth was actually like; in fact, she learned what birth was like from watching *A Baby Story* on TLC:

> CHARLENE: I watch . . . *[A] Baby Story*, [in] which they take you straight through labor and delivery. And some people have [epidurals], some people don't, and you can watch cesareans. . . . I found it to be more helpful . . . to watch those shows than those awful videos they showed during the classes.
>
> INTERVIEWER: So, how would you say that those [affected] you? Did they give you any expectations or ideas about what you wanted?
>
> CHARLENE: Yeah, I think probably I got more the idea that . . . what I saw during those shows is definitely in line with actually what occurs, where what I saw at the class, I mean it just didn't seem like it could be really that way.

It is clear that Charlene believes these shows are representative of how birth occurs in U.S. hospitals, but she may not be aware of the subtle framing that goes on in the shows that make women appear weak and dependent on maternity care providers or of the overrepresentation of interventions and c-sections.

Women, then, increasingly have questionable information about labor and birth and common interventions, while at the same time medical decision making is being pushed down to patients. Pushing patients to be the ultimate deciders in medical care transfers the risk of the decision from the provider to the woman. It is commonplace, in fact, for physicians across medical specialties to delegate decision-making responsibility about care to patients, who might then be more likely to assume responsibility for a bad outcome. In essence, this shift is another attempt to avoid blame for bad outcomes. Although this shift in decision making has been written about in the medical literature, it is not generally seen as a movement in the patients' best interest. In fact, ACOG's Ethics Committee suggests that using the informative model of decision making, in which physicians strictly provide information to the patient but the patient makes medical decisions, "raises concerns about physicians' protecting themselves rather than working in the best interests of their patients."[33] Further, scholars of ethics question whether such a model of decision making is consistent with informed consent if physicians do not give a recommendation for treatment.[34]

Thus, while maternity providers push decision-making responsibility onto patients, most women's sources of information are biased and not evidence-based, and few women understand the risk of interventions and c-sections, even women who plan to have a c-section.[35] Maternity providers, because of their training, have more and better information than do women about the risks of various birth interventions. In any situation where there is asymmetric information—that is when one decision maker has more information than another decision maker—the person with the lesser amount of information cannot make decisions rationally.[36] In other words, rational decisions require full information, something few patients have. What this means is that although women are asked to make decisions, they must still rely on what they believe maternity providers want them to do, even if the maternity providers' preferences does not come in the form of an official "recommendation." It is easy to see how under these conditions, maternity providers can influence a woman's decision by their presentation of risk. Maternity providers expect women to make decisions about how to give birth, but their presentation of risk has a heavy influence on a woman's decision. Therefore, women tend to make the decisions the way the maternity providers would like them to make the decision, but without maternity providers' bearing the responsibility—the woman made the choice. Further, if a woman *chooses* a c-section, then the provider may also not be culpable if she is injured by the c-section.

An example of how this type of interaction happens is demonstrated in the following interview excerpt, in which physician Lois Timberlake discusses how choice is presented to women who for a medical reason must hasten birth either through an induction of labor or a scheduled c-section. She tells me, "We're just more likely [now] instead of saying, 'We have to go through the exercise of labor,' we're much more likely to say, 'Look. We've got a 10 percent chance of this working. Do you want go through labor or not?'" Maternity providers present "choices," but it is also clear that the way they present the risks guides women's decisions.

Physicians understand this power they have to persuade women to have a c-section by how they present risk. Physician Geneva Spalding spoke about the vulnerability women have during labor and the asymmetrical information that exists between laboring women and maternity providers:

> I do feel that a physician is in a position that the woman trusts. This is a very vulnerable time. So the woman will do [what the physician says], unless she feels very empowered and is very well educated. . . . When you have no knowledge of medicine, you really depend on that physician to guide you.

This idea of how maternity providers counsel or provide information to patients was noted repeatedly in the interviews as an important element of how patients make choices. Some maternity providers candidly told me that they could make patients do anything they want just by changing how choice and risk are presented. Here are a few examples:

> It's very easy to get someone to agree to have a c-section when you say to them, "Your baby is OK now, but there is no guarantee that if the strip remains this way that I can guarantee that everything is going to be OK later, and I think it's best to take the baby out and then you don't need to worry." [It is] sort of rare that [the] mother is going to say to you, "No, I'd rather wait and see if my baby has a problem later on." So the presentation of the decision making is a little bit skewed, and people are very skittish. (Physician Maggie Rust)

> We were taught [that] . . . we were supposed to use the best judgment we can to make that decision, yet . . . not every woman can spontaneously deliver a baby so . . . we're going to make that judgment. Who is safe to do a forceps or vacuum [on] and who should have a c-section? The monitor is not perfect, but she is OK, and she is OK to labor, and we will make that judgment. Now we know that we are not perfect, and . . . [if] I'm really good I may be able to tell you 90 percent of the time, but not 100 percent of the time, and I'm not willing, I know that limitation. *And when I explain that limitation to you, to make it only fair that you know it, you tend to opt for the c-section.* (Physician Allen Homan; emphasis added)

What this means, taken to the logical extreme, is that a perfect vaginal birth outcome cannot be guaranteed; when this information is shared with women, they are said to *choose* c-sections. The question becomes: are the risks of c-section accurately presented?

Similarly, physician Eric Kraemer mentions how women can be persuaded to make certain decisions:

> You can talk a woman into or out of [c-sections]. And that's true of most of the things, whether hysterectomy, surgery, and that's what's so important about doctors' realizing the trust that the patients have placed in them is a real sacred trust. And we have to be very careful [not] to abuse that. I think that people who might abuse it don't abuse it on purpose and

think about it, as they know best. And that's the biggest—one of the big-gest—faults many of us can be accused of in the medical world: we know best. And, therefore, the whole concept of informed consent is all in how you pitch it.

In other words, maternity providers can heavily sway women to make the "right" decision.

Informed Consent in Labor and Birth

This ability of maternity providers to sway women's decisions, intention-ally or unintentionally, leads directly to a discussion of informed consent in medicine. I quote here information provided by the American Medical Association and directed at physicians:

Informed consent is more than simply getting a patient to sign a written consent form. It is a process of communication between a patient and physician that results in the patient's authorization or agreement to un-dergo a specific medical intervention. In the communications process, you, as the physician providing or performing the treatment and/or pro-cedure (not a delegated representative), should disclose and discuss with your patient:

- The patient's diagnosis, if known;
- The nature and purpose of a proposed treatment or procedure;
- The risks and benefits of a proposed treatment or procedure;
- Alternatives (regardless of their cost or the extent to which the treatment options are covered by health insurance);
- The risks and benefits of the alternative treatment or proce-dure; and
- The risks and benefits of not receiving or undergoing a treat-ment or procedure.

In turn, your patient should have an opportunity to ask questions to elicit a better understanding of the treatment or procedure, so that he or she can make an informed decision to proceed or to refuse a particular course of medical intervention.

This communications process, or a variation thereof, is both an ethical obligation and a legal requirement spelled out in statutes and case law in all 50 states.[37]

When reflecting upon what informed consent should involve, it is clear that informed consent in maternity care is lacking, and this observation is supported by much research.[38] Ethicist Veronique Bergeron writes of modern labor and childbirth, "Because childbirth no longer belongs to birthing women, the latitude of autonomous choice they possess is determined by those who now own the proper conduct of childbirth. Women are invited to exercise unlimited autonomy within the limited range of choices presented to them by the medical profession."[39] Researchers Habiba and colleagues in a 2006 article published in *BJOG* phrased this concern in the following way: "Rather than expressing a free, informed choice for caesarean delivery, [women] may become trapped between the obstetricians' attitudes, lack of opportunities for nonmedicalised vaginal birth and media-publicized fashionable trends featuring vaginal delivery as unsafe, archaic, disfiguring and ultimately socially unacceptable."[40]

In fact, most consent forms are generalized to cover all maternity care procedures women may encounter during labor and birth, with the exception of anesthesia and c-sections, both of which have separate consent forms.[41] The general form is signed before or upon admission to the hospital. Some hospitals do not have formal consent forms for women in labor and birth. Rather, women imply consent by seeking treatment at the hospital. Scholars question whether informed consent can be obtained when a procedure's risks are not clearly understood.[42] The idea of informed consent is also complicated by the question of whether women can adequately consent to procedures during labor, especially when they are in pain.[43] Further, even when the forms list benefits and risks of interventions, physicians may not discuss the risks enough during the informed consent discussion, a problem mentioned by physician Jacob Chism:

> People are busy on both sides. Patients are busy. Physicians are busy. I think discussions are happening about risk and benefits, but I think they are very brief, relatively superficial, and there is not a lot of persuasion going on. If somebody says to me, "I want an induction done." "Well, you know, it is going to increase your [chance of] c-section, you may [be] induced for many hours. It may not necessarily be in your best interest to do this electively." "Yeah, but I really want it because my mother is going to be in town." "OK. Fine. Let's just do it." And that's the extent of the conversation. . . . I think there is a difference between informed consent and just simple due diligence. I might be obligated to tell somebody the risks, but not necessarily in a way that I'm engaging and trying to persuade

them one way or the other. I'm just running off a checklist saying, "OK, this is associated with this. Oh, you still want it? OK." Well, leave it at that and move on.

Combining this lack of informed consent with the findings that many women lack information about interventions such as continuous CTG, Pitocin augmentation, amniotomy, induction, epidurals, and c-sections, it becomes difficult to see how true choice is present in modern maternity care. In essence, scholars argue that the notion of choice has been confined to women's choice among medical interventions and does not take into account the social and cultural context within which choices are presented to women.[44] As Holly Goldberg argues in her 2009 article published in the *Journal of Perinatal Education*, "Patient participation in informed decision making . . . is dependent on the availability and accessibility of choice and alternatives."[45]

Conclusion

Framing choice in reproductive care must be comprehensive. The rhetoric of choice has been focused on a woman's right to choose to deliver by c-section, even though it is questionable that many women are demanding this choice. Yet it is not as common to think of choice in terms of a woman's right to choose to deliver a breech baby or twins vaginally, to choose to attempt a vaginal birth after a c-section, or to refuse labor interventions in the hospital. Women may not have these choices because maternity providers, hospital administrators, malpractice insurers, and reinsurers may not be willing to allow her to labor in these situations.[46] It is clear from this situation that what drives choice is the attempt to protect the baby from a bad outcome, but even more so to protect the maternity provider from liability, key values that are integrated into a woman's care when she is pregnant. In short, birth is not about a woman's choice.

Organizations constrain greatly women's choices in labor and birth. Most women are not well educated about interventions or the risks of c-sections. Yet the trend is for health care providers to ask patients to make decisions, while at the same time guiding them toward c-sections or interventions, like inductions, ultrasounds, continuous CTG, that lead to c-sections. It is easy to see in such a situation how the way maternity providers present the decision is so important, and as can be seen in my earlier analyses in this book, many health care providers' views are greatly colored by their perception that they will be blamed for bad outcomes. Under these conditions, informed consent cannot happen, and this has been pointed out in the ethical debate about maternal request for elective c-section.[47] In a similar way that scholars of reproductive justice have pointed out that reproductive "choice" is not possible without social and economic justice, I suggest that "choice" in labor and birth is also not possible due to organizational constraints.

Conclusion

A Roadmap for Change

I have demonstrated in this book that the escalating c-section rate cannot be explained by blaming women or maternity providers. Women are not choosing to have c-sections and physicians are not performing c-sections because they believe it is the best health option. Rather, organizational change and constraints are responsible. Hospital administrators, ACOG, courts, malpractice insurers, and reinsurers have defined c-sections as the best practice *to protect themselves and maternity providers from blame in the case of a bad outcome*. Further, hospital administrators and risk managers have put in place control systems by way of protocols to align the decisions and actions of maternity providers and women with the organizational goal of reducing liability threats. These control systems define appropriate care for women in labor and birth and limit the decisions and actions of care providers. Yet most of these protocols are not based on overwhelming scientific evidence of improved health outcomes. Quite the opposite—they are contributing to the escalating c-section rate, which threatens the health of women and babies. The c-section epidemic is an organizational paradox: women's health is at risk, health care costs are soaring, and babies are not protected.

Any effort to resolve the c-section epidemic requires organizational solutions. For example, a study that examined how best to decrease inductions and scheduled c-sections before thirty-nine weeks gestation found that when physicians were educated about the risks of birth before thirty-nine weeks, the rate of pre-thirty-nine-week inductions and c-sections did not decrease significantly.[1] The most important factor leading to a decrease in inductions or c-sections before thirty-nine weeks was the presence of a hospital policy prohibiting them. In other words, it is fanciful to think that relying on educating individual maternity providers about interventions will lead to the best medical decisions for their patients. These individuals are actors within an organizational context that greatly affects their behavior.

We can make sense of this by remembering Weber's notion of explanatory understanding.[2] That is, we cannot understand social trends without understanding the motives that lie beneath and are causing the trends. It is important to understand that maternity providers have agency in these situations—especially obstetricians who make the decision about inductions and c-sections—and that this agency is at the root of the social trends to induce labor and to perform c-sections. Yet one must understand why maternity providers make the decisions that lead to these trends. For example, educating physicians about risks of different interventions, such as delivery before thirty-nine weeks or c-sections, will not stop the trend if lack of education is not causing their decisions in these situations. Physicians generally know it is better for women to deliver vaginally after thirty-nine weeks, but they are also concerned about *liability*. In other words, it is concern about liability that drives many of their decisions, not lack of education. Maternity providers' notions of risk affect their decisions, and thus to enact change, *organizations* must change their guidelines and protocols and meaningful malpractice reform must happen.[3] The answer to the c-section epidemic must go beyond blaming individuals and move toward *solutions* to resolve this irrational organizational paradox.

Change is possible. The c-section epidemic is a human creation. Humans created it, and humans can destroy it. Below I group solutions to the c-section epidemic as follows: immediate changes that individuals can enact, changes that organizations can make, and large-scale societal changes, which are the most difficult to enact and will take time and concerted effort to accomplish. I do discuss individual changes even though I have argued that individual change alone cannot resolve this paradox. Consistent with the arguments in this book, for real change to happen organizations must change. Yet organizational change takes time, and the women who are being injured by the practices in question are not in control of the organizations. Until organizations change and while organizations are changing, I feel it important to give women and maternity providers ideas about what they can do now to help solve the c-section epidemic.

Immediate Solutions for Women Who Plan to Give Birth

SOLUTION 1: *Women should take independent childbirth education classes*

Many women do not take childbirth education classes, and those who do typically take them at hospitals.[4] Hospital-based childbirth education classes have been shown to normalize interventions and c-sections.[5] Women should seek out independent childbirth education classes to learn about the empirical evidence around birth practices and interventions. Directories to find these types of classes can be found through Birthing from Within (http://www.birthingfromwithin.com/), BirthWorks (http://www.birthworks.org/), BrioBirth (http://www.briobirth.com/), International Childbirth Education Association (http://www.icea.org/), and Lamaze International (http://www.lamaze.org/). Women who take these classes will be more informed about labor and birth, and this step can immediately help reduce their chance of having a c-section, largely because women who take such classes are more knowledgeable about and can therefore avoid interventions that increase their risk of c-section.

SOLUTION 2: *Women should seek out maternity providers and hospitals with low intervention and c-section rates*

Because VBAC rates are so low and because the risks from c-sections snowball over time and with each additional c-section, women should try to prevent a first c-section.[6] One way to do this is to choose carefully one's maternity provider and place of delivery. Most women will have to seek information on intervention and c-section rates of hospitals and maternity providers by calling hospitals and obstetrical practices and asking for the data. Hospital c-section rates are sometimes available on state websites, typically under the department of public health, but only Massachusetts and New York mandate that hospital, but not provider, c-section rates be published. Women should ask about rates of labor induction, labor augmentation, and c-section and whether continuous CTG is used routinely to monitor a baby in labor. Women should also ask providers how long they would allow a pregnancy to extend before suggesting an induction, and whether the provider recommends ultrasounds at the end of pregnancy for all women. Further, women should consider using a midwife or family physician as a maternity provider because these providers have lower c-section rates than do obstetricians, and also because they tend to have attitudes more conducive toward less interventionist birth than do obstetricians.[7]

SOLUTION 3: *Women should use evidence from childbirth classes to inform their birth experiences, refuse interventions that are not evidence based, and insist on practices that are evidence based*

For example, women should refuse ultrasounds in the last month of pregnancy unless maternity providers can demonstrate a high-risk condition that would require such strict surveillance because women who have ultrasounds during the last month of pregnancy are more likely to have c-sections.[8] Women should also refuse induction or a scheduled c-section because it is suspected that their baby is macrosomic. We know that delivering suspected macrosomic babies by c-section does not improve birth outcomes.[9] Further, low-risk women should refuse continuous CTG monitoring, nonmedically indicated inductions, routine augmentation, and having their membranes artificially ruptured (which increases pain and c-section risk but does not shorten the second stage of labor). On the other hand, women should insist on being monitored intermittently, using movement during labor to help deal with pain and to move labor along, and having the choice to proceed with VBACs, vaginal twin deliveries, and vaginal breech deliveries. Perhaps most important, women should share with their maternity providers their preference for a vaginal birth. Maternity providers need to hear this from women. Women should write birth plans in which they make clear their preferences for labor and birth and should share this plan with her maternity providers during prenatal appointments and at the hospital during labor and birth.

SOLUTION 4: *Women should hire birth doulas to accompany them during birth*

Evidence suggests that women who are attended in birth by doulas have shorter labors, less interventions, and lower rates of c-section.[10] A birth doula meets with a woman a few times during pregnancy to get a sense of what the woman expects from birth and to work with her on a plan to help her attain the birth she desires. During labor and birth, a birth doula gives the woman encouragement and support, and this care has been shown to improve outcomes. Women can find a doula by searching the DONA International directory at http://www.dona.org/.

SOLUTION 5: *Women should consider giving birth in freestanding birth centers or at home*

Entering the hospital means that women are subject to protocols and interventions that are not evidence based but rather protect the hospital in the case of a bad outcome. Staying at home or giving birth at a freestanding birth center gives pregnant women more decision-making opportunities and control over how they give birth. Evidence suggests that when low-risk women give birth at home or a birth center, outcomes are just as good if not better than for low-risk women who give birth in a hospital and rates of interventions and c-sections are lower.[11] Encouraging women to give birth at home or in a freestanding birth center is also in the interest of the U.S. health care system, as giving birth at home or in a birth center costs less than giving birth in a hospital.[12]

Women can find a list of freestanding birth centers by consulting the American Association of Birth Centers (AABC) at http://www.birthcenters.org/. Unfortunately, birth centers are not available to all women. According to the AABC, there are only 215 birth centers in the United States.[13]

Finding a home birth midwife may also be difficult. Because the certification and licensure laws of home birth midwives vary by state, there is no national directory of home birth midwives. To find a midwife who attends home births, women can start by examining the state-by-state directory of Birthing Naturally at http://www.birthingnaturally.net/directory/. Women can also contact independent childbirth education teachers or doulas in the area and ask if they know of any home birth midwives. Because not all states certify and license home birth midwives, women have to be diligent in seeking out midwives who are qualified to attend birth. Karen Bayne, a birth doula and childbirth educator with Gentle Balance Birth in Northampton, Massachusetts (http://www.gentlebalancebirthnorthampton.com/), shared a set of questions she gives women to ask home birth midwives they are considering hiring to attend a birth:

- What does the midwife say about *contraindications* for home birth? (If she says "none," that is not a good answer.)
- What does the midwife say about *transferring* patients to the hospital during labor if it is not going well? (Has she done this before? Is she willing to talk about it)
- Does the midwife accompany her patient *into* the hospital? If she cannot due to legal reasons, how does important information travel from home to hospital?

- Which hospital does she send patients to? Is that a place you feel comfortable going?
- What kinds of equipment does she bring that would be helpful if you need medical help but not at a hospital? (Sutures for stitching? Infant resuscitation equipment?)

Women should also ask for references from other patients of the midwife. Women should feel comfortable with the answers they receive from the midwife and from the references before hiring a home birth midwife.

The trend of out-of-hospital births is picking up. A 2011 study documented a 20 percent increase in women giving birth at home.[14] But to make home birth a viable option for more women, health insurance companies should be required to cover home birth expenses. Only New York and Washington State require that health insurance companies cover home birth expenses, and until this is required in all states, home birth is a luxury available only to women who live in these states, those who live in other states but are successful in seeking reimbursement from their health insurer, or those who can pay the $3,000–$5,000 out-of-pocket expense.

SOLUTION 6: *Women who suffer side effects from c-sections, whether physical or psychological, should litigate for damages, especially if they feel the c-section was unnecessary*

This is not an optimal solution, as it just perpetuates the use of malpractice lawsuits in a way that is not useful to society. But until significant change happens in the malpractice system, this may be the only way that women can get the attention of organizations like ACOG, hospitals, malpractice insurers, and reinsurers and force them to promote evidence-based practices that improve the outcomes for women and babies. If financial risk is the defining measure for ACOG, hospitals, and insurers, this is one way to enact change.

Immediate Solutions for Maternity Providers

SOLUTION 1: *Maternity providers should be up front with women about birth risks and the notion that sometimes things go wrong in pregnancy, labor, and birth even with the best of care*

This type of discussion should happen when physicians and midwives provide routine gynecologic and prenatal care to women. Admitting the unpredictability of a natural process is uncomfortable. Women may not want to face the reality that sometimes births do not turn out perfectly, and providers may not like admitting that they cannot guarantee perfect outcomes. But this is a necessary first step. Here are two examples of how maternity providers could talk about this reality. Physician Andrew Robinette tells me, "[If I ruled the world] I would tell people that it's not up to us how their baby comes out to a certain degree." Midwife Candace Whitt's point is the same: "Universally I will say to patients sometime in their pregnancy, 'Hey, listen, we can do everything right, and still this can go wrong. That's how life works out.' And I think that message has to get out there. It's got to come out of your mouth." This approach needs to be emphasized more in medical education. It goes without saying that as medical knowledge has advanced, more lives have been saved. But there is a limit to what medicine can do. Maternity providers need to be taught to be humble and to share with patients that they cannot solve every medical problem or prevent every bad outcome.

SOLUTION 2: *Maternity providers should provide women with Cochrane Review articles as a way of promoting evidence-based practices in pregnancy, labor, and birth*

The Cochrane Collaborative publishes very useful "plain language summaries" of their reviews, and women at a middle-school reading level should be able to understand them. Maternity providers should distribute these articles to all women who seek prenatal care. They should also use these articles as a springboard for discussion with women about the advantages and disadvantages of labor and birth interventions.

SOLUTION 3: *Physicians should voice their concerns to ACOG about the increasing c-section rate and about non-evidence-based protocols*

ACOG is a physician-based organization. It does not exist without physicians, and it listens to physicians. Physicians should tell ACOG their concerns not only with liability, which many already do, but also with the c-section epidemic and with non-evidence-based practice guidelines. Physicians should tell ACOG officials that they are unwilling to support the promotion of protocols that are not evidence based and that contribute to the escalating c-section rate. Physicians can write letters to ACOG, attend ACOG meetings, or call their ACOG district representative (a list of districts and representatives is available at http://

www.acog.org/About_ACOG/ACOG_Districts). If enough physicians indicate to ACOG their concern with non-evidence-based practices, ACOG will have the incentive to better integrate evidence-based practice into practice bulletins, which will, in turn, protect physicians who practice evidence-based care from being held responsible for bad birth outcomes that are not due to medical error. ACOG practice guidelines are often used to establish a standard of care that a physician is expected to provide to patients. Particularly, if the practice guidelines are evidence based, maternity providers should be able to argue in court that they were following guidelines that are established based on the best scientific evidence available.

Organizational Solutions

SOLUTION 1: *Hospitals, obstetrical medical practices, and maternity providers should be required to publicly disclose their intervention and c-section rates*

Part of the reason women lack information about labor and birth is that data about hospitals' and providers' intervention and c-section rates are not readily available. Requiring that these rates be published online on the states' public health websites and mandating that maternity providers distribute this information to women when they seek prenatal care would be a start. Currently New York and Massachusetts are the only states that mandate hospitals disclose their c-section rates. As part of another research project, I have collected hospital c-section rates from many different states with varying degrees of success. For example, although California typically charges a fee to access these rates, the California Public Health Department sent this information free of charge when I made an academic inquiry. On the other hand, Maryland refused to disclose hospital c-section rates upon my request, citing privacy concerns. Further, I was forced to file a Freedom of Information Act request to obtain Connecticut's hospital c-section rates (even though I am a resident of Connecticut and teach at a Connecticut college). In short, these rates are not accessible in all states. Midwife Joyce Linville tells me of the deterrent effect on c-sections that this disclosure would have: "If somebody's c-section rate were common knowledge, that in itself would provide some incentive to wanting to do the changes."

SOLUTION 2: *Hospital-based informed consent should cover all birth intervention separately (oxygen masks, Cytotec, Pitocin, continuous CTG, epidurals, episiotomy, forceps, vacuum extraction, etc.)*

Women should be given all of the information on birth and labor interventions during pregnancy, and maternity providers should take time to go over this information carefully with patients. Women will then be better prepared to consent to interventions during labor and birth. For example, research shows that when women are given information about and then asked to decide which monitoring technique they prefer, intermittent auscultation or continuous CTG, they are more likely to choose intermittent auscultation.[15] This is an indication that women make rational decisions about care and interventions when they are provided with evidence about the intervention and outcomes.

SOLUTION 3: *ACOG practice guidelines and hospital protocols should reflect scientific evidence of improved outcomes*

For example, continuous electronic fetal monitoring detects some babies who are struggling, but, with a 99.8 percent false positive rate, it usually identifies as struggling, babies who are perfectly healthy, many who end up being unnecessarily delivered by c-section. Intermittent fetal monitoring should become the norm for most women, especially because outcomes are just as good with intermittent monitoring with a Doppler as with continuous CTG.[16] The routine use of continuous electronic fetal monitors should be stopped. As it is, the tracings from the electronic fetal monitors are seen as necessary to maternity providers because the strips produced are used in court cases involving bad birth outcomes to suggest when interventions should have been done. Physician Rosemary Steel eloquently talks about this problem: "It's weird. Continuous fetal monitoring is one way that people are afraid that we might miss something. But it is also one of the bigger reasons why we get sued. So it's like, we make all these interventions to try to help, but we end up just hurting ourselves the other way around." If all hospitals and maternity providers were to agree to stop the routine use of continuous CTG together, then the liability issue connected to its use would instantly go away. Further, the heavy use of inductions, Pitocin, epidurals, and the artificial breaking of women's amniotic sacs should be questioned because these interventions are not based on evidence of improved fetal or maternal outcomes. On the other hand, technologies that are useful in evaluating how the baby is tolerating labor—the pH scalp sample, fetal pulse oximetry, and STAN—and technologies that may help women achieve a vaginal birth—vacuum extraction and forceps—should be promoted.

A number of existing organizations have the goal of making labor and birth better for women and babies, and they should be brought into the conversation in terms of establishing protocols and standards of care for labor and birth. For example, BirthNetwork National (http://www.birth-network.org/), Childbirth Connection (http://www.childbirthconnec-tion.org/), Coalition for Improving Maternity Services (http://www.motherfriendly.org/), International Cesarean Awareness Network (http://www.ican-online.org/), International Childbirth Education Association (http://www.icea.org/), and Lamaze International (http://www.lamaze.org/) all advocate for changes that promote the health of women and babies. ACOG and hospital administrators should listen to these groups.

SOLUTION 4: *Hospital administrators, malpractice insurers, and reinsurers should not be allowed to ban VBAC attempts, vaginal breech deliveries, or twin deliveries*

Women should have all of these options. Empirical evidence does not suggest that the routine use of c-sections in these situations improves outcomes.[17] We need to recognize that denying a woman the option of a vaginal delivery means that she is forced to have a c-section, which is a serious infringement on a woman's right to control what happens to her body. VBAC is relatively safe, certainly no more dangerous than a woman's first vaginal delivery, and catastrophic uterine rupture is exceedingly rare. Remember that half of all c-sections are repeat c-sections, and, thus, increasing VBAC attempts would drastically lower the c-section rate in the United States. Over half of all pregnant women with a prior c-section would like the opportunity to have a vaginal birth, and this percentage may well increase with concerted public health messages that suggest the relative safety of this mode of delivery.[18] ICAN and other groups that support birth options after c-section should be given serious public attention to spread their message. As Physician James R. Scott, editor in chief of the official journal of ACOG, *Obstetrics and Gynecology*, in his June 2010 editorial, wrote, "What level of risk is acceptable, and who decides? Currently, hospitals, insurance companies, and plaintiff attorneys decide or strongly influence whether VBAC is an option."[19] But should these *organizations* decide women's choices? Further, routine c-sections for twins and for babies presenting in a breech position is also not supported by evidence of improved outcomes. Routine c-sections from babies presenting in breech position is based on the flawed findings of the Term Breech Trial.[20] This trial also affected vaginal twin deliveries because one of the twins presenting in a breech position is a very common occurrence.

SOLUTION 5: *Medical schools should require obstetrics residents be trained on how to facilitate VBACs, vaginal breech deliveries, and vaginal twin deliveries, and how to use forceps and vacuum extraction to facilitate vaginal birth*

Because few physicians now see these types of birth, they do not know what to expect, and the dread of liability and bad outcomes looms large in their minds. Thus, to save vaginal birth opportunities for women, there must be a concerted effort to train new obstetricians in VBAC and vaginal twin and breech births and in the use of forceps and vacuum extraction. Many maternity providers have these skills, but if we wait too long, these technical skills will exist only in the hands of those who have retired. As Doctor Jacob Chism tells me:

> Now the skill set to do [vaginal births], the tolerance for tracings that are not perfect, the ability to do operative vaginal delivery using forceps or vacuum, those are all gone for a whole generation of ob-gyns, and everybody in the under-forty-five set struggles with these things now and doesn't have the skills to do it. So, if you look at the graph of section rates over the years, when have they ever gone down significantly? Never. We've just been able to maintain [the rate]. So, I'd be a little surprised if we get down under 30 percent down the road.

I am not as pessimistic as Doctor Chism, because I talked to many providers who have these skills. But Chism's assessment suggests the importance of medical schools requiring residents to learn these skills.

SOLUTION 6: *Hospitals should employ doulas and more nurses so that women have one-to-one care during labor and birth*

As mentioned earlier, evidence suggests that women who are attended by doulas and have one-to-one care have shorter labors, less interventions, and lower rates of c-section.[21] Thus there should be a public health initiative to increase the nursing staff in maternity care and also to publicly fund doula programs. As it is, usually the only women who have doulas at their births are women who have the economic resources to hire them privately.

Most private health insurance companies do not pay for doula care, and most hospitals do not provide doulas free of charge. Insurance companies should recognize the positive financial outcome of doulas—hiring a doula is much cheaper than paying for a c-section.

Nurses could also play more of a doula role if they had only one woman to monitor in labor and also if something were done to relieve their excessive documentation responsibilities. Physicians are aware that having nurses devoted to standing at the bedside of women is part of a solution to the escalating c-section rate, as discussed by physician Geneva Spalding: "It's a shame, because we're not [employing more nurses]. We're saving money on one side, but we're not on the other side. I mean, absolutely it makes a big difference when you have a nurse [who] can now give 100 percent time."

SOLUTION 7: *Hospitals should mandate that every c-section be reviewed, and c-section should once again be defined as a quality measure*

As I pointed out in chapter 2, maternity providers recall when c-sections were reviewed and how that influenced their practice. They were less likely to jump quickly to a c-section because they did not want to be publicly exposed as having performed an unnecessary procedure. Bringing mandatory c-section reviews back would undoubtedly bring c-section rates down. Perhaps mandatory c-section reviews could be made a requirement of hospital accreditation. This speaks to a larger issue of the patient safety movement, which insists that c-section not be a measure of quality. This must be changed.

SOLUTION 8: *Insurance companies should experience-rate physicians such that malpractice insurance rates reflect past experience and current practice*

Those physicians without any prior lawsuits should have lower rates than those with a prior malpractice suit. Physicians should also have their premium based on the number of births they attend. As it is, obstetricians pay the same premium regardless of the number of births they attend and the number of lawsuits filed against them. The practice of not tying premiums to number of births attended also discourages obstetricians from practicing part time, as they must pay the same malpractice insurance premium as those obstetricians practicing full time, but they do not have the same number of patients to spread out the cost of the premium. This was cited as a problem by a number of obstetricians in my interviews.

Long-Term Societal Solutions

SOLUTION 1: *Reform the malpractice system in the United States*

Reforming the malpractice system would go the furthest to solving the c-section epidemic. Birth advocacy organizations like Childbirth Connection also see the importance of malpractice reform to improving maternity care in the United States.[22] It should be pointed out that not only does the current medical malpractice system lead to a higher c-section rate, it also does not meet the needs of many patients. For example, it is well documented that most patients who suffer from medical negligence do not receive legal reprieve and that malpractice settlements and awards are more closely linked to the severity of disability than to the degree of medical negligence.[23] Maternity providers are very clear that the malpractice system in place now does not work from their perspective. Physician Jack Bianco sums up what I heard from most providers with the following statement:

> [The rising c-section rate is due to] four words: lack of tort reform [a type of malpractice reform]. That's it. . . . You want to question anyone, . . . anything . . . the top 99 percent will all relate to that. . . . I'm a provider. You can talk to whomever you want [who] sits inside a building deciding on public policy. . . . You can talk to one hundred people, one thousand people [who] don't presently [deliver babies], but if you talk to people [who] do [deliver babies], that's the reason. That's it. Done deal. Done. Slam dunk.

Maternity providers are frustrated, and they shared with me the structural problems they feel are embedded in the current malpractice legal system. For example, part of their frustration is that it is not possible for anyone to always be perfect, including maternity providers. Providers feel the pressure of the impossible demand by society that they never make a mistake. This was mentioned repeatedly in the interviews I conducted with maternity providers, such as physician Philip Burgin:

> This is a tough world to be in because we have to be perfect. When you think of any other human endeavor—your job [as a college professor] . . . can you be wrong? Of course you can be wrong. CEOs of companies, they can be wrong. . . . I mean presidents . . . can be wrong in deciding to go to war. . . . We can't be wrong. . . . Let's say we actually make a mistake.

Let's say I, as a doctor, didn't see something, didn't figure out something fast enough, didn't do something I should have done, OK. Am I human? Am I going to practice for twenty-five years and not make a mistake? . . . I didn't intend to do this, but it happened. I was too sleepy; I hadn't read the book; whatever. I made a mistake. . . . You can do that, right? . . . And [are] your health and house and livelihood at risk when you say that? . . . And is it even reasonable that society would expect that of its doctors. We're human, and yet that's the standard we're held to—perfection.

Physician Andrew Robinette concurs when he says, "There's not perfection in anything. So why—somebody does their best 99.9 percent of the time and 0.1% of the [time], even if they made a mistake—why should it cost them their reputation?"

To complicate matters, birth has a particular liability conundrum—not every bad outcome is tied to bad care, and bad things sometimes happen when everything is done correctly. As physician Jack Bianco tells me, "The problem is [that] every bad baby does not necessarily mean that we made a mistake."

Building on this idea is the fact that many providers feel that they are being sued in part because families with disabled children may simply not have enough money or resources to adequately care for a disabled child. This is important to understand—maternity providers are concerned about the infants. It is not *just* liability. They typically go into medicine because they want to help people. This concern about families' needs for money to care for disabled children was mentioned by a number of maternity providers. Here are a few examples:

What we really need to realize is that in some outcomes what happens is that, you've got a baby who's going to need advanced support for the rest of its life, and the patient [and] the parents are suing because financially they don't have the wherewithal to support the child. (Midwife Rita Morey)

I'm out there; I'm a normal human being. Meaning, you know, anyone who makes less than $25 million a year, whatever . . . and I have a baby that has a bad problem, that's going to need a lifetime of care. . . . Insurance won't pay for it, not in any noble way. . . . So what do I do? The only thing I can do is [to] try to claim fault so that someone pays for it. I'm going to sue in a heartbeat. I might. You might. I wouldn't say I wouldn't do it. (Physician Jack Bianco)

Another frustration maternity providers talk about is having medical evidence evaluated and their behavior judged by people who are not medical professionals. Physician Maggie Rust articulates this concern:

> One of them I knew ... actually went to trial and she's like, "It's not a jury of my peers that are all on the jury, I'm trying to explain medical empirical evidence to them, and they're looking at the poor mom who's crying. So, how can they judge my job when they're not a jury of my peers?" They don't understand my practice. They understand the sympathies of the mother. So, you also feel like it's stacked against you, too.

In short, providers feel the current medical liability system is not in their or their patients' interest.

I would like to suggest a possible solution to the malpractice problem that would address these structural issues. The renowned surgeon and writer, Atul Gawande, in an essay in the *New Yorker*, highlighted this solution. Gawande discusses an alternative approach to dealing with compensation for medical injuries.[24] He based his solution on how vaccination injuries are currently handled.[25] Although millions of children are protected by vaccinations, about one in every ten thousand children who receives a vaccination will experience negative side effects. In the 1980s, when these vaccination injuries were being heavily litigated and plaintiffs were winning huge awards, vaccine prices increased and some drug manufactures abandoned the production of vaccines—the risks were seen to outweigh the benefits. When vaccines came in short supply, Congress acted. On October 1, 1988, the National Childhood Vaccine Injury Act was passed. This act created the National Vaccine Injury Compensation Program, which established a pool of money through a seventy-five-cent surcharge on all vaccines to compensate vaccination-injury victims regardless of whether the injury was due to medical error. If a patient's family is not satisfied with the payment, they can sue under the traditional tort system. But, in fact, most families do not seek other relief, and the program is seen as hugely successful, having paid out $1.5 billion to injured patients between 1988 and 2005.[26]

A similar system should be developed for birth injuries because promoting the health of women and children is also a public health issue. Congress could become just as concerned with the historic rise in the c-section rate and establish a similar fund for birth injuries. This would be a no-fault system, one that is advocated by many of the obstetricians I interviewed and also by ACOG.[27] An expert panel would come up with a list of possible birth injuries. Anyone who experiences a birth injury on the list is compensated, regardless of whether a medical error was committed. If a board of medical experts determines malpractice, then an additional award would be made to the family and the offender would be dealt with in ways that protect patients from a pattern of medical errors. Families would also have the ability to seek redress through the current system, just as patients with vaccination injuries can. Recall that few of those families take this step.

In fact, Florida and Virginia have implemented programs that share some similarity to this vision: the Florida Neurological Injury Compensation Association, created by the Florida legislature in 1988, and the Virginia Birth-Related Injury Compensation Program, established by state legislation in 1987.[28] Both programs remove the requirement of negligence from compensation for a birth injury. However, they are quite restrictive on which injuries are compensated. The injury must be severe enough to cause substantial physical *and* mental disability, *and* must be due to oxygen deprivation or mechanical injury. Both programs require most patients to work through the program in the case of a birth injury.[29]

These programs are administrative malpractice solutions and were developed to deal with a perceived liability crisis. The goal was to move claims for compensation of children with severe neurological impairments from the traditional courts and provide hospitals and maternity providers immunity from malpractice lawsuits. Both programs are funded primarily through fees paid by hospitals and maternity providers and are largely seen as a success. However, they have not reduced the c-section rate. Both states have c-section rates above the national average. In 2011 (the most recently available data), while the national c-section rate was 32.8 percent, Florida's rate was 38.1 percent and Virginia's was 34.1 percent.[30]

My proposal is different from the NICA and BIP programs in a few respects, all aimed at addressing the c-section epidemic. First, all children with physical *or* mental birth injuries would be compensated, regardless of whether there was oxygen deprivation or mechanical injury. This would be an outcomes-based program, and such a program would be considered, according to Siegal, Mello, and Studdert, a targeted social insurance program, or a form of social insurance that is available to only very specific people, in this case those born with birth injuries.[31] I would advocate that a *social* program is exactly what we need to address the rising c-section rate. All children with negative birth *outcomes* should be cared for, regardless of how the injury occurred. Second, the goal of the program would not be only to resolve the liability crisis, but also, and more importantly, to lower the c-section rate and, as a result, improve the health of women and babies. Third, medical courts would be a part of the process of finding medical errors. To avoid the problem that patient advocates identify with such a system—that medical providers protect one another—medical experts would be appointed for a given time with their only job being to research cases in which medical error is alleged. One model would have many or all of the experts being physicians with academic appointments, because academics are generally more steeped in the empirical literature than are physicians who are strictly clinicians. These experts would be bound to use the most rigorous scientific evidence available. The medical experts would work for the government, not for either the plaintiff or the defendant. Physician Andrew Robinette talked about the role of medical boards: "Let's have medical courts. Let us have a lawyer and a doctor and a judge, all who have medical training in some way shape or form. . . . They are really a jury, in a sense, of your peers."

Having such a program would have immediate effects. First, the documentation requirements of nurses would almost necessarily lessen if an outcomes-based birth injury compensation fund were implemented, and lessening these requirements would surely allow nurses to spend more time with women in labor. Second, physicians would not be as likely to practice defensively and the c-section rate would be lowered. Not only would lowering the c-section rate be a defined goal of the program, but also because all birth injuries would be covered and a board of medical experts would decide negligence, the liability anxiety expressed by maternity providers would necessarily lessen. Maternity providers spoke about how a no-fault malpractice system would allow them to practice less defensively. For example, physicians Jack Bianco and Andrew Robinette tell me:

And there are ways around it. . . . No-fault auto insurance killed the big litigant industry. . . . We should have some version of that for doctors, some sort of no-fault insurance payout for cases that are reasonably reviewed where there wasn't fault. Of course, people shouldn't be allowed to get away with doing dumb things, and they shouldn't practice bad medicine. (Physician Jack Bianco)

Well, my idea was, when you get pregnant, [you] throw two hundred bucks in the kitty. It's an insurance plan. And then babies who are [damaged] are compensated [through the funds that women and their families have paid into the insurance plan]. . . . Everybody said, "OK, look, not everything goes right with a patient, with the pregnancy. Mom can die—pregnancy is the most dangerous thing you do . . . and babies can die." . . . In most of the cases the doctor wasn't sitting there and planning . . . to do some malpractice—I'd rather be home or . . . I want to be sleeping. . . . They were really, really trying to do their best. (Physician Andrew Robinette)

In short, this solution to how to deal with negative birth outcomes would leave maternity providers feeling less vulnerable and, thus, allow them to deliver better care. The c-section rate would almost certainly decline as a result.

SOLUTION 2: *The United States should move toward a system that promotes midwifery care and out-of-hospital birth*

A general move toward a less medicalized system of birth would also help to solve the c-section epidemic. Birth advocates often focus on the Netherlands when they are looking for optimal models of birth.[32] In this discussion I draw from an analysis of this model and ideas of how it could be applied to the United States set forth by De Vries and colleagues in their 2009 chapter titled "The Dutch Obstetrical System: Vanguard of the Future in Maternity Care."[33] The Dutch model defines a pregnant woman as having either a physiological (low-risk) pregnancy, in which case midwives or general practitioners oversee her care, or a pathological (high-risk) pregnancy, in which case gynecologists oversee her care. In the Netherlands, 80 percent of women begin their prenatal care with a midwife and 6.5 percent with a general practitioner, and about 30 percent of women give birth at home.[34] Outcomes in the Netherlands are better than outcomes are in the United States—the U.S. infant mortality rate is twice the infant morality rate in the Netherlands (six per thousand live births compared to three per thousand live births).[35]

The Dutch system has important features that lead to these outcomes. First, the health care system is state organized and includes an "Obstetrics Indications List," which carefully distinguishes between physiological (low-risk) and pathological (high-risk) pregnancies.[36] Women who have a physiological pregnancy must seek care from a midwife or general practitioner. Women seek care from gynecologists only when they meet a condition on the list. Second, the midwives, gynecologists, and general practitioners work well together and are given clear guidelines of collaboration by the government, insurance companies, and professional organizations.[37] Third, there is political support in the Netherlands for midwifery and home birth.

The United States should focus on this type of model because it prioritizes women's and babies' health. We should promote midwives and family physicians as the care providers of low-risk women. If these women need to transfer to obstetricians because of a problem that develops in their pregnancies, this should be seamless. Further, women who are defined as low risk—the vast majority of women—should be encouraged to give birth at home or in birth centers. This is probably the biggest obstacle to such a system in the United States because ACOG does not support home birth, and home birth midwives have been criminalized in some states.[38] In addition, there is a lack of freestanding birth centers in the United States. In essence, many physicians do not believe in or support home birth or birth center practices, and many women lack access to such care.

It is also crucial under such a system for midwives and physicians to collaborate because women may need to transfer care. If they do need to transfer to a physician for care, there needs to be continuity in care and respect for the patient. This is especially true if the transfer of care occurs when the woman is in labor. Communication must be facilitated among providers, and a woman's transfer of care, whether from provider to provider in the hospital or from home or birth center to hospital, must be seamless. This is often not the case in the United States, especially when women transfer from a home birth to the hospital, where the woman and the midwife may be treated in a hostile manner. In some states midwives may even not be allowed to accompany their patients to the hospital because the hospital will not grant midwives privileges and because midwives fear legal consequences for being identified as practicing home birth midwifery. This problem would largely be solved if all states licensed home birth midwives. There is a movement to accomplish this goal: the Big Push for Midwives (http://pushformidwives.org/). As of this writing in February 2013, twenty-seven states have passed legislation to authorize the practice of certified professional midwives (CPMs) or home birth midwives.

De Vries and colleagues in their 2009 chapter have a very interesting idea on how structural change could happen in the United States. They highlight a contradiction between the cultural focus in the United States on health, wellness, and protecting babies and a highly medicalized system of labor and birth in which women and babies are subjected to drugs and non-evidence-based practices that might cause harm. These authors conclude, "Birth activists should seize on the contradiction and use it as a wedge to open a policy conversation about the costly, impersonal, and dangerous way of birth in the United States."[39]

Change Must Happen

Change is essential for the health of babies and women and for the viability of the U.S. health care system. Maternal mortality in the United has increased by over 40 percent over the past two decades, from 12/100,000 live births in 1990 to 21/100,000 live births in 2010.[40] The effect of c-sections on maternal mortality rates is well documented in the United States and in some individual states, particularly California, a state that has put money and other resources into documenting and trying to stem the rise in maternal morality.[41] Several maternity providers expressed a concern about the rising maternal mortality rate and its relationship to the soaring c-section rate. Physician Jeffrey Starling says, "The other potential cost [of the rising c-section rate] is in maternal mortality rising, maternal mortality due to placenta accreta, which worries me a lot and, . . . even in [the] best [of] hands, women can still die with placenta accreta because it's such an extraordinarily dangerous thing to have." Physician Allen Homan makes a similar point: " I think we have the same maternal death rate now as Belarus, so I think we're doing something wrong. Our maternal death rate is rising. . . . [And that is because of] c-sections." Likewise, physician Jacob Chism says, "Well, I think [in the next five to ten years] we'll have the data to show . . . [increasing] maternal mortality due to hemorrhage, placenta previa, placenta accreta, all the things associated with repeat cesareans. Then we're going to see a significant pop in maternal mortality in this country. . . . There is already some data out of California that is suggesting that that is the direction we're headed."

If women's increasing risk of dying does not grab the public's attention, perhaps the money we are spending on unnecessary c-sections will. Recall that c-sections cost almost twice that of vaginal deliveries, and in 2008 there were 1.4 million cesarean surgeries performed at a cost of about $8.7 billion.[42] Researchers suggest that $5 billion could be saved on an annual basis by reducing the c-section rate to 15 percent.[43] I heard about this problem from maternity providers, like midwife Jill Wayland—"We're spending so much money unnecessarily on all this intervention [and c-sections]. It's outrageous. In obstetrics it's really outrageous. . . . And then we have other people who can't get care and die unnecessarily because we're spending money ridiculously"—and physician Jack Bianco—"The economics of c-sections being more expensive, and costlier, and making us less money are totally off the table because people are afraid of $100 million lawsuits." In other words, we all must commit to resolve the irrational paradox of the c-section epidemic. This is important to women's and babies' health and to our economy.

Conclusion

Combined, the solutions I have presented would go a long ways toward solving the c-section epidemic and making birth safer. Alone, each is a step in the right direction, and many can be accomplished by individual actions. We all can make positive changes, and that is why I will end this book on an optimistic note.

Change has begun, although slowly. The c-section rate actually declined from 32.9 percent in 2009 to 32.8 percent 2010, the first decrease in the trend since 1996, and held steady at 32.8 percent in 2011.[44] This is really something to celebrate. Further, the Joint Commission, an organization that accredits health care organizations, including hospitals, developed a new set of Perinatal Care Core Measures in 2010. Starting on January 1, 2014, hospitals with 1,100 or more births per year will be required to report on the Perinatal care measure set, including the c-section rate.[45] Hospitals with less than 1,100 births may choose to report on these measures.[46] Although this requirement of mandatory reporting for hospitals does not start until 2014 and does not include all hospitals, it is still a step in the right direction.

Good news is also on the horizon if the Affordable Care Act (i.e., "Obamacare") is not dismantled. For example, health insurance companies will not be allowed to charge women higher insurance premiums than men, to use "pregnancy" or "past c-section delivery" as a condition to deny women insurance coverage, or to deny coverage for maternity care, all things that are legal without the new legislation.[47] This shows the effect that laws can have on improving reproductive health for women.

Efforts to recognize the importance of reducing the c-section rate can also be accomplished through government action and a focus on maternal health. I see these changes as an indication that organizations can respond to the irrational paradox of a high c-section rate and make changes that will improve the health of women and babies.

Methods Appendix

In this book, I rely on in-depth interviews of maternity providers and post-partum women as the primary source of data. I conducted interviews with maternity providers between 2007 and 2010 over the phone and in person. All of the maternity providers practice in Connecticut with the exception of one physician and two midwives who practice in other northeastern states. I used snowball sampling to identify maternity providers to interview; I asked each maternity provider whom I interviewed to recommend other maternity providers to contact, and maternity providers sometimes sent e-mails to colleagues suggesting they contact me about being interviewed for the study. I also attended a Connecticut American College of Obstetricians and Gynecologists meeting and an obstetrical practice meeting where I described my research to attendees, distributed information sheets about the research, and asked for their participation. Further, I sent an e-mail solicitation to Connecticut midwives through the American College of Nurse–Midwives. Trinity College's Institutional Review Board approved the study.

Table A.1 presents the breakdown of maternity providers by occupation and gender. In total I interviewed fifty maternity providers: twenty-five physicians (50 percent), twelve midwives (24 percent), and thirteen labor and delivery nurses (26 percent). I oversampled physicians because physicians make the decision to perform a c-section; thus I thought it important to talk to many physicians to see how they come to that decision. All of the nurses and midwives I interviewed are female. This is not surprising because nearly all labor and delivery nurses (97.2 percent in 2008) and certified nurse-midwives (99 percent in 2005) in the United States are women.[1] The physicians in my study have more gender diversity, with 36 percent being female and 64 percent being male. Female obstetricians are slightly underrepresented in my data, as the latest data available suggest that in 2010 49 percent of physicians in the United States specializing in obstetrics and gynecology are women.[2]

Table A.1. Maternity provider characteristics

Gender		
Physicians		
Female		36%
Male		64%
(N)		(25)
Midwives		
Female		100%
(N)		(12)
Nurses		
Female		100%
(N)		(13)
Race/ethnicity		
Physicians		
White		96%
Black		0%
Hispanic		2%
Asian		2%
(N)		(25)
Midwives		
White		100%
(N)		(12)
Nurses		
White		100%
(N)		(13)
Years licensed		
Physicians		
Mean		19.48
Range		3–31
(N)		(25)
Midwives		
Mean		8.75
Range		1–19
(N)		(12)
Nurses		
Mean		18.38
Range		6–37
(N)		(13)

The maternity providers are white with the exception of one Latina physician (2 percent) and one Asian physician (2 percent). Although I would have preferred a more racially diverse sample of maternity providers, because midwives, physicians, and labor and delivery nurses in the United States are overwhelmingly white, my sample reflects this demographic truth. The American Medical Association (AMA) has the most comprehensive information on physician characteristics. In 2010, the most recently available data from the AMA, race is known for 82 percent of physicians specializing in obstetrics and gynecology in the United States.[3] For those physicians whose race is known, 71 percent of physicians specializing in obstetrics and gynecology are white, 11 percent are Asian, 9 percent are Black, 7 percent are Hispanic, and 1 percent are of another race.[4] Nurses and midwives are less racially diverse than are obstetricians. In 2008, the most recently available data, 83.2 percent of registered nurses in the United States are white.[5] Midwives in the United States are overwhelming white, with 95.2 of certified nurse–midwives listing white as their race.[6]

Physicians in the study range in years since completion of their graduate education from three to thirty-one years, with an average of 19.48 years. Midwives range in time since first license from one to nineteen years, with an average of 8.75 years. Nurses range in time since first license from six to thirty-seven years, with an average of 18.38 years.

I was interested in finding out why maternity providers think the c-section rate is increasing, and how they feel about that increase. Maternity providers all understood that the rate has increased over time. I didn't speak to any maternity provider who disputed the trend. The interviews were semi-structured. I first asked, "What is your overall feeling about the cesarean section rate increase?" I then followed up with a very general question: "What do you feel are the primary reasons for this increase?" The bulk of the data for the book come from maternity providers' answers to this question. Maternity providers varied in how long they took to answer this question. Some took just a few minutes, whereas others took upward of thirty minutes. After they answered this question, I then continued with the following: "I have made a list of reasons that are cited for the increased c-section rate. This list comes from various sources, both academic and lay. Some reasons are fairly controversial. I will read each reason on the list, leaving out the causes you have already mentioned, and would like you to discuss with me, from your perspective, whether each contributes to the increase in the c-section rate." The reasons I listed were:

- Cesarean delivery by maternal request
- Increased maternal age
- Increased rates of obesity
- Increased prevalence of multiple births
- Decreased likelihood of operative vaginal deliveries
- Increased use of epidural anesthesia
- Increased incidence of labor induction
- Increased use of continuous electronic fetal monitoring
- Increased use of Pitocin to augment labor
- Increased ability to diagnose fetal distress
- Decreased likelihood of vaginal birth after cesarean section
- Economic incentives of hospitals
- Hospital liability concerns
- Economic incentives for physicians
- Physician liability concerns
- Impact of medical literature
- Physician scheduling convenience

My analysis of women's birth experiences is based on eighty-three interviews that were conducted between June and December of 2010 with postpartum women at a Connecticut tertiary care hospital where 3771 women gave birth in 2010. Four research assistants, two with bachelor's degrees and two in their last year of undergraduate study, conducted the interviews. The interviewers were trained and supervised by the author of the book. The Institutional Review Boards of Trinity College and the hospital both approved the interview questions and research protocol. The hospital stipulated that the interviewers could not interview anyone under eighteen years of age or anyone who did not speak fluent English. In collaboration with the postpartum nurse manager of the hospital, we developed a protocol whereby on the days they went to the hospital, the interviewers attempted to interview all women who had given birth the day before and who were also eighteen years of age or older and fluent English speakers. Overall, we interviewed eighty-three women.

Table A.2 contains demographic information for the women interviewed. In terms of race, 61.4 percent of the women are white, 21.7 percent are Black, 8.4 percent are Hispanic, 6.0 percent are Asian, and 1.2 percent identified as multiracial or some other race. One woman declined to give her race. These percentages do not reflect perfectly the racial characteristics of women who gave birth in the hospital in 2010. White (48.3 percent),

Black (15.2 percent), and Asian (4.4 percent) women are overrepresented in our sample, while Hispanic women (28.1 percent) and women who are mixed race or another race (4.0 percent) are underrepresented. The underrepresentation of Hispanic women is almost certainly due to our not interviewing women who were not fluent speakers of English.

About two-thirds of the women shared household income information (four women declined to share their annual household income and twenty-three women reported being unsure of their annual household income). Almost one-third of the women report annual family income of at least $100,000, with 16.9 percent reporting annual household income between $100,000 and $149,000 and 15.7 percent reporting annual household incomes of $150,000 or higher. The largest share of women (26.5 percent) fell in the $50,000 to $99,000 annual household income category. Only 8.4 percent of women reported annual household income of less than $50,000, although, given the education date reported below, it seems safe to assume that likely many of the women who did not report income were from the lower-income brackets.

In terms of education, nearly two-thirds of the women interviewed have a bachelor's (32.5 percent) or graduate degree (32.5 percent). Fewer women have a high school degree or less (14.4 percent) or some college but less than a bachelor's degree (20.5 percent). Women range in age from nineteen to forty-one, with an average age of 30.4 and a median age of 31. The age distribution of women who gave birth in the hospital in 2010 is similar to our sample, with the acknowledgment that we lack the youngest women giving birth. For women who gave birth in the hospital in 2010, the mean age was 29.2, the median age was thirty, and the range in age was from fourteen to forty-eight.

My goal for these interviews was to understand what women expected their births to be like and what they were actually like. To that end, the main question the interviewers asked was, "Would you share with me the story of your labor and birth? The more details you share with me, the more it will help us to understand your birth experience." The interviewers were trained to prompt women with questions about plans for birth, such as strategies for pain medication and preference for vaginal birth or c-section. They also prompted women when appropriate to find out whether they had their labors induced or augmented, received analgesic pain medication, or had other interventions. They followed up with questions on the woman's attitude toward the birth experience—"What is your general feeling about the labor and birth? Was it a positive experience?"—and

Table A.2. Postpartum women characteristics

Race/ethnicity	
White	61.4%
Black	21.7%
Hispanic	8.4%
Asian	6.0%
Other/mixed race	1.2%
Declined	1.2%
(N)	(83)

Income	
Less than $50,000	8.4%
$50,000–$99,000	26.5%
$100,000–$149,000	16.9%
$150,000 or more	15.7%
Declined	32.5%
(N)	(83)

Education	
High school or less	14.4%
Some college	20.5%
Bachelor's degree	32.5%
Graduate degree	32.5%
(N)	(83)

Age	
Median age	31.0
Mean age	30.4
Age range	19–41
(N)	(83)

Note: Table percentages may not add to 100 percent because of rounding error.

expectations about the birth—"During your pregnancy, did you have an expectation or wish about what your labor and birth would be like?" They ended the substantive questions with, "Do you wish anything had gone differently during this labor and birth? And, if so, what do you wish had gone differently?" Further, they asked women who had repeat c-sections whether they had been interested in having a VBAC and whether one had been offered to them.

Notes

Notes to the Introduction

1. All names used in the book are pseudonyms.
2. Jain and Dudell 2006.
3. A doula provides nonmedical physical and emotional support to a woman during labor and birth. Doulas are typically hired by women who plan to give birth in a hospital and who want to maintain control over their labor and birth. However, doulas may also attend home births or may be hospital employees who attend laboring women, sometimes free of charge and sometimes for a fee. Health insurance companies in the United States do not pay for doulas to care for women during labor. Having a doula attend a woman's birth has been shown to significantly decrease a woman's labor time, to decrease the likelihood of interventions and c-section, and to increase the woman's positive feelings about the birth. See Hodnett et al. 2011; McGrath and Kennell 2008; Simkin and O'Hara 2002; Kennell et al. 1991; Klaus et al. 1986.
4. Rozen, Ugoni, and Sheehan 2011; Landon et al. 2006.
5. Hamilton, Martin, and Ventura 2012.
6. I owe a great debt to other sociologists and anthropologists who have studied reproduction and drawn attention to reproduction as a scholarly topic, including Jeanne Flavin (2009); Wendy Simonds, Barbara Katz Rothman, and Bari Norman (2007); Elizabeth Armstrong (2003); Monica Casper (1998); Robbie Davis-Floyd and Carolyn Sargent (Davis-Floyd and Sargent 1997; David Floyd 1992); Brigitte Jordan (1997); Faye Ginsburg and Rayna Rapp (1995); and Ann Oakley (1986).
7. In this book, the term "fetus" will be used for gestations under twenty-eight weeks, the defined age of viability, and "baby" will be used for gestations at or over twenty-eight weeks. The exception will be if the term "fetus" is used in a specific study. In such a case, I will adopt the use of the term as well.
8. Modified or new items on the 2003 birth certificate form include: mother's and father's race (multiple race identification); mother's and father's

education (highest degree earned); cigarette smoking levels before and during pregnancy; method of delivery including fetal presentation and trial of labor prior to cesarean section; pre-pregnancy weight, weight at delivery, and height (to calculate BMI); congenital anomalies; fertility therapy; whether the mother received WIC food for herself during pregnancy; infections during pregnancy; maternal morbidity; breast feeding; and the principal source of payment for the delivery.

9. Childbirth Connections 2012.

10. Martin et al. 2012; Declercq et al. 2006.

11. Hamilton, Martin, and Ventura 2012.

12. Based on statistics presented in Declercq et al. 2006.

13. Ibid.

14. Based on statistics presented in ibid.

15. Ibid.

16. The description of the c-section surgery is based on that presented in Boston Women's Health Book Collective 2008.

17. Declercq et al. 2006.

18. Martin et al. 2012.

19. Declercq et al. 2006.

20. A Pinard stethoscope, a trumpet-shaped device placed on the woman's abdomen, can also be used to monitor the baby's heartbeat, although maternity providers have told me that they very rarely if ever see a Pinard being used anymore. It has been shown that if a woman is monitored with a continuous electronic fetal monitor during admission to the hospital, she is more likely to have a c-section than if she is monitored with a Doppler unit or a Pinard stethoscope. See Devane et al. 2012.

21. Declercq et al. 2006.

22. Declercq et al. 2006 report a 41 percent induction rate, whereas Martin et al. 2012 report an induction rate of 23.4 percent. The inductions rates differ, I suggest, because induction is likely being underreported in the birth certificate data used by Martin et al. 2012. Declercq et al. 2006 use survey data in which women self-report whether they were induced.

23. Declercq et al. 2006.

24. Alfirevic, Devane, and Gyte 2006.

26. American College of Obstetricians and Gynecologists 2009.

27. Ibid.; Alfirevic, Devane, and Gyte 2006.

28. Alfirevic, Devane, and Gyte 2006.

29. Ibid.

30. Ibid.

31. Ibid.
32. Ibid.
33. Ibid.
34. Hofmeyr and Lawrie 2012.
35. Hendrix et al. 2000.
36. Alfirevic, Devane, and Gyte 2006.
37. Clark and Hankins 2003; Blair and Stanley 1993.
38. Alfirevic, Devane, and Gyte 2006.
39. Grimes and Peipert 2010; Nelson et al. 1996.
40. Ibid.
41. Declercq et al. 2006.
42. Alfirevic, Devane, and Gyte 2006.
43. Declercq et al. 2006.
44. Ibid.
45. Ibid.
46. Halpern et al. 1998.
47. Ibid., 2109.
48. Boston's Women Health Collective 2008, 179.
49. Declercq et al. 2006.
50. Smyth, Alldred, and Markham 2007.
51. Declercq et al. 2006.
52. Rollins and Lucero 2012.
53. Singata, Tranmer, and Gyte 2010.
54. Declercq et al. 2006.
55. Ibid.
56. Ibid.
57. Ibid.
58. Gherman et al. 2006; Sokol, Blackwell, and American College of Obstetricians and Gynecologists 2003.
59. Sokol, Blackwell, and American College of Obstetricians and Gynecologists 2003.
60. Ibid.; Sacks and Chen 2000; Ecker et al. 1997; Perlow et al. 1996.
61. Rouse and Owen 1999.
62. Declercq et al. 2006.
63. Boston Women's Health Book Collective 2008.
64. Declercq et al. 2006.
65. MacDorman, Menacker, and Declercq 2008.
66. Kuklina et al. 2009; Villar et al. 2007; Deneux-Tharaux et al. 2006.
67. Deneux-Tharaux et al. 2006.

68. Villar et al. 2007.
69. MacDorman et al. 2008.
70. Declercq et al. 2008; Knight et al. 2008; Declercq et al. 2007; Whiteman et al. 2006.
71. Osborne et al. 2012; Clark and Silver 2011; Landon 2010; Daltveit et al. 2008; Gray et al. 2007; Yang et al. 2007; Usta et al. 2005.
72. Grady 2008.
73. Callaghan, Creanga, and Kuklina 2012.
74. Ibid., 1034.
75. The literature on risk of pelvic floor damage resulting in urinary incontinence and/or pelvic organ prolapse is voluminous but weak. There has not been a prospective randomized trial (that is women have not been randomly assigned to have a c-section or vaginal birth) with long-term follow up comparing incontinence and prolapse in women who have c-sections to women who give birth vaginally. Further, most studies are not able to separate out the effects on incontinence of pregnancy, number of children born, and method of delivery, nor do they have common definitions about what constitutes incontinence or prolapse. Taking this into account, what the existing empirical literature suggests is that vaginal birth may contribute to incontinence compared to c-section in the first year after birth; however, one year after giving birth there is no difference in urinary incontinence between those women who delivered by c-section and those women who delivered vaginally Ekstrom et al. 2008; Press et al. 2007; Glazener et al. 2006; Fritel et al. 2005; McKinnie et al. 2005; Faundes, Guarisi, and Pinto-Neto 2001; Wilson, Herbison, and Herbison 1996; McKinnie et al. 2005. And, although some studies indicate that the most extreme injury of a weakened pelvic floor, pelvic organ prolapse, is more common in women who have given birth vaginally than women who have had a c-section, the evidence shows in general that the risk of uterine prolapse is slight—few woman under age 60 have pelvic organ prolapse—and that prolapse is also related to factors other than mode of birth, such as smoking, family history, weight, and number of pregnancies. Larsson, Källen, and Andolf 2009; Rortveit et al. 2007; Hendrix et al. 2002; Samuelsson et al. 1999.
76. Hansen et al. 2008; Salam et al. 2006; Alexander et al. 2006.
77. Walsh et al. 2011; Clark and Hankins 2003.
78. Glantz 2011.
79. Boyle et al. 2012; Fuchs and Gyamfi 2008.
80. Fuchs and Gyamfi 2008.
81. World Health Organization 1985.

82. Data for this figure are taken from three sources: Taffel, Placek, and Liss 1987; Centers for Disease Control and Prevention 1995; Martin et al. 2012. It is also important to note that the c-section rate is highest for Black women, a fact that has yet to be well explained. See Martin et al. 2012.
83. World Health Organization 1985.
84. World Health Organization 2012a.
85. Ibid. It is important to recognize that in the United States Black women are more than 2.5 times as likely to experience maternal mortality than are white women. See Centers for Disease Control and Prevention 2012. In short, there is incredible racial disparity in maternal mortality rates in the United States.
86. Catlin et al. 2008.
87. Sakala and Corry 2008.
88. Podulka, Stranges, and Steiner 2011.
89. Sakala, Delbanco, and Miller 2013.
90. Dumont et al. 2001.
91. The documentary *Dead Mums Don't Cry* gives a particularly poignant picture into how c-sections can save the lives of women, and how women die from their lack of access to this surgery. See Quinn 2005.
92. See United Nations 2012.
93. Tang et al. 2006; Patel et al. 2005; Ben-Haroush et al. 2004; Lin et al. 2004; Young and Woodmansee 2002; Aron et al. 2000.
94. Declercq et al. 2006.
95. For example, see McCourt et al. 2007.
96. Kalish, McCullough, and Chervenak 2008; Gossman, Joesch, and Tanfer 2006; Declercq, Menacker, and MacDorman 2005; Gamble and Creedy 2000.
97. Nilstun et al. 2008; Young 2006.
98. Weaver, Statham, and Richards 2007.
99. Gamble and Creedy 2000.
100. American College of Obstetricians and Gynecologists 2008.
101. Bergeron 2007; Habiba et al. 2006.
102. Lagrew and Adashek 1998; Tussing and Wojtowycz 1993; Tussing and Wojtowycz 1992; Turner, Brassil, and Gordon 1988.
103. Tussing and Wojtowycz 1994; Rock 1993.
104. The literature on whether malpractice fear affects maternity providers' decision about performing c-sections is mixed. Some find that it does affect c-sections. See Yang et al. 2009; Murthy et al. 2007; Brown 2007; Benedetti et al. 2006; Tussing and Wojtowycz 1997; Localio et al. 1993; and Rock 1988. Others find no relationship. See Sloan et al. 1997; Baldwin et al. 1995. Still others find that the effect is short-lived or weak. See Dranove and Watanabe

2010; Grant and McInnes 2004; and Dubay, Kaestner, and Waidmann 1999. Insightful summaries of the malpractice environment and the historical context of crises have been written about by other scholars, including Kachalia, Choudhry, and Studdert 2005; and Studdert, Mello, and Brennan 2004.
105. Goodrick and Salancik 1996.
106. Giddens 1971.
107. Ibid.
108. Ibid.
109. Weber and Shils 1949.
110. Collins 1986.
111. Martin 2003.
112. Resource dependence theory suggests that survival is the ultimate goal of organizations and that organizational survival is threatened by lack of autonomy and uncertainty. Organizations proactively attempt to resolve uncertainty and lack of autonomy to ensure survival through a number of strategies, including avoiding uncertainty, changing the organization, changing the environment, or some combination of the three. See Palmer 1983; Pfeffer and Salancik 2003; and Pfeffer and Nowak 1976. Because, according to this theory, organizations exist within a network of other organizations, including suppliers, customers, rivals, and regulators of the organization, uncertainty and lack of autonomy can come from any of these organizations. Further, to the extent that market changes cause uncertainty for the organization's survival, macroeconomic changes may threaten the organization. See Pfeffer and Salancik 2003.
113. Anderson 2012.
114. See Shortell 2000; and Robinson 1999 for interesting discussions of the increase in competitive pressures on hospitals.
115. Stevens 1989.
116. Ibid.
117. Ibid.
118. See, for example, discussions in Starr 1982; and Shi and Singh 2012.
119. Liebhaber and Grossman 2007; and author's computations taken from the Health Tracking Physician Survey (Center for Studying Health System Change 2008).
120. Shi and Singh 2012.
121. Sloan and Chepke 2008.
122. Ibid.
123. Klagholz and Strunk 2009.
124. See Jaffee 2001 for a good discussion of organizational responses to external uncertainty.

125. Benson 1977.
126. Gillum and Bello 2011.
127. The notion that administrators put in place organizational structures is discussed by many organizational theorists, including Pfeffer and Salancik 2003; and Cyert and March 1963. Although they approach this topic from different perspectives, they share a commonality in suggesting that organizational structures constrain the behavior of individuals within organizations.
128. Timmermans and Berg 2003 make a compelling argument that evidence-based medicine and randomized clinical trials have become the gold standard in the health care field. They explore the politics of standardization in medicine—who controls standardization and how it changes medical care. Similarly, I suggest that c-sections have become the "gold standard" of care for women in birth and that this definition also has political roots.
129. I understand that medical sociologists and anthropologists would approach this topic quite differently and that my using an organizational framework takes a different approach. I value the approach of medical sociologists and anthropologists and their research and believe that examining the important role organizations play in birth can add new understanding to the topic by using a different and innovative approach.
130. I interviewed maternity providers practicing in Connecticut, except for two providers who practice in Massachusetts and one who practices in New Jersey.
131. See http://www.cochrane.org/ (accessed April 15, 2011).
132. Martin et al. 2012; Declercq et al. 2006.

Notes to Chapter 1

1. Klagholz and Strunk 2009 (emphasis added).
2. Sloan and Chepke 2008.
3. Ibid.
4. Ibid.
5. Klagholz and Strunk 2012.
6. Gherman et al. 2006; Mello 2006; Clark and Hankins 2003; Sokol, Blackwell, and American College of Obstetricians and Gynecologists 2003; Blair and Stanley 1993.
7. See, for example, Baker 2005; and Centner 2008.
8. Klagholz and Strunk 2012.
9. Jena et al. 2011.
10. Greve 2009.

11. Klagholz and Strunk 2012.

12. Ibid.

13. Ibid.

14. See, for example, Baker 2005; and Centner 2008.

15. This is thought to be the result of both high costs of litigating malpractice suits and litigating attorneys' reluctance to assume any cases that do not have a good chance of a high settlement or judgment. See Sloan and Chepke 2008.

16. Ibid., 61.

17. Author's calculations from National Practitioner Data Bank public data set available from U.S. Department of Health and Human Services 2010.

18. Author's calculations using data available for purchase from *Medical Liability Monitor*.

19. Sloan and Chepke 2008, 59.

20. State of Connecticut Insurance Department 2009.

21. Sturdevant 2011, 1.

22. Mello 2006.

23. Ibid.

24. Klagholz and Strunk 2012.

25. Mello 2006; Hay 1992.

26. Hay 1992.

27. Shea et al. 2008.

28. Shi and Singh 2012.

29. Sloan and Chepke 2008.

30. Ibid.

31. Ibid., 10.

32. Jena et al. 2011.

33. Mavroforou, Koumantakis, and Michalodimitrakis 2005.

34. Localio et al. 1991 also find that most victims of medical errors are not compensated.

35. Sloan and Chepke 2008.

36. Brennan, Sox, and Burstin 1996.

37. Xu et al. 2008.

38. Friedrich 1963, 16.

39. Ibid.

40. In 2001, the most recent comparison I could find, there were 350 percent more malpractice claims filed per 1,000 population in the United States than in Canada, although the actual claims paid in the United States were somewhat lower than claims paid in Canada. See Anderson et al. 2005.

41. Declercq et al. 2006.

Notes to Chapter 2

1. Ransom et al. 2003.
2. See Jaffee 2001 for a particularly cogent discussion of this issue and how human control has been incorporated into various organizational theories.
3. Simon 1976; Cyert and March 1963.
4. Simon 1976; March and Simon 1958.
5. March and Simon 1958.
6. Ritzer 2004.
7. Wright et al. 2011.
8. Kesselheim and Studdert 2006.
9. Ibid.
10. Kohn, Corrigan, and Donaldson 2000.
11. Clark et al. 2011.
12. See, for example, Abuhamad and Grobman 2010; Greenberg et al. 2010; Clark et al. 2008a; Clark et al. 2008b; Pearlman and Gluck 2005.
13. Pettker et al. 2009. Clark et al. 2008a report a decrease in c-section rates after implementation of patient safety protocols (from 23.6 percent in 2005 to 21 percent in 2006), but this has not been reported by other researchers; further, I remain skeptical of this claim because it is based on a one-year decrease, which could be due to any number of factors other than patient safety protocols.
14. Silver 2010; Flood et al. 2009; Knight et al. 2008.
15. See Timmermans and Berg 2003 for an interesting study on the political dimensions of standardization of medical care. In their terms, the type of standardization to which I refer is "procedural standardization," which specifies processes. They argue that we need to get beyond analyzing just the positive and negative effects of standardization to understand better the historic roots and the political issues involved.
16. Ibid.
17. Stevens 1989.
18. Ibid.
19. Ibid.
20. Ibid., 331.
21. Kesselheim and Studdert 2006.
22. Statistics taken from Dekker 2012.
23. Hannah et al. 2000.
24. Glezerman 2006.
25. For criticisms of this study, see ibid.; Kotaska 2011; Kotaska 2004.

26. Glezerman 2006.
27. Hannah et al. 2004.
28. Hofmeyr, Hannah, and Lawrie 2010; American College of Obstetricians and Gynecologists 2006.
29. Schutte et al. 2007.
30. Glezerman 2006, 24.
31. Hofmeyr, Barrett, and Crowther 2011.
32. Martin et al. 2012; Martin et al. 2011.
33. Hofmeyr and Kulier 2012.
34. Ibid, 2.
35. GE Healthcare 1997.
36. Macones et al. 2008.
37. Pettker and Lockwood 2008.
38. Ibid.
39. Ibid.
40. Ibid.
41. Matthews 2000.
42. Alfirevic, Devane, and Gyte 2006.
43. Ibid.
44. Ibid.
45. Clark et al. 2009b.
46. See especially ibid. See also Rooks 2009 for a critique of this perspective.
47. See Kotaska, Klein, and Liston 2006 for this study. See Clark et al. 2009b for information on the low-dose oxytocin protocol advocated by the patient safety movement.
48. Clark et al. 2009b advocate for a team approach in oxytocin administration and increased authority for nurses to determine appropriate Pitocin use. For example, they write, "Our combined experience in reviewing literally thousands of cases involving adverse outcomes or litigation tells us that with rare exception, in disagreements between nurse and obstetrician regarding the aggressiveness of oxytocin administration, the experienced nurses is generally correct" (35.e4).
49. An intrauterine pressure catheter is a catheter that is placed alongside the baby to measure the strength and length of a woman's contractions.
50. Janis 1971.
51. Shaw-Battista et al. 2011 find that a collaborative practice with midwives and physicians can provide excellent care of women and produce positive outcomes.
52. Clark et al. 2009b, 35.e4.

53. Clark and Silver 2011.

54. "Apgar" refers to how a baby's health is assessed after delivery. Five character-istics of the baby are assessed, and for each characteristic the baby receives a score of 0, 1, or 2, with 0 being a low score. The characteristics measured are: appearance (skin color/complexion); pulse (pulse rate); grimace (reflex to stimulation); activity (muscle tone); and respiration (breathing). The scores are combined at one minute after birth and again at five minutes after birth. A combined score of 7 or above is considered normal. It is common for the scores to be given in succession, such as a nurse telling a new parent that the baby had Apgars of 7 and 9, meaning that the baby's Apgar score was 7 one minute after the birth and 9 five minutes after birth. This score was developed by Virginia Apgar in the 1950s and is seen as having revolutionized infant care because it not only puts a focus the baby, but it guides very specific ways of assessing the baby, although some criticize the score for being too compartmentalized and not fo-cused on the general health of the infant. See Gawande 2006 for an interesting history of the development of the score and its advantages and disadvantages.

55. Wagner et al. 2011.

56. Ibid.

Notes to Chapter 3

1. Davis-Floyd 1992.

2. As an aside, there is no evidence that giving women oxygen improves fe-tal outcomes (Fawole and Hofmeyr 2003). Yet this intervention clearly is something that bothered Cecelia; according to *Cochrane Review* authors, "so deeply entrenched is its use in clinical practice that healthcare workers al-most intuitively administer oxygen at the first suspicion of fetal distress" (2).

3. Declercq et al. 2006 report that 99 percent of women received at least one ultrasound during pregnancy.

4. Ibid. See Taylor 2008; Mitchell 2001; Sandelowski 1994; Petchesky 1987 for a discussion of the social implications of ultrasound technology.

5. Sokol, Blackwell, and American College of Obstetricians and Gynecologists 2003; Sacks and Chen 2000; Acker, Sachs, and Friedman 1985.

6. Irion and Boulvain 2009; Alsunnari et al. 2005; Sacks and Chen 2000; Ecker et al. 1997; Johnstone et al. 1996.

7. Gherman et al. 2006.

8. Foad, Mehlman, and Ying 2008.

9. American College of Obstetricians and Gynecologists 2002.

10. Walsh et al. 2011.

11. Ibid.

12. National Center for Injury Prevention and Control 2011.

13. Little et al. 2012.

14. Ibid.

15. Parry et al. 2000.

16. Declercq et al. 2006.

17. Abuhamad and ACOG Committee on Practice Bulletins 2008.

18. Ibid.

19. Ibid.

20. Melamed et al. 2010.

21. Declercq et al. 2006.

22. Little et al. 2012; Bricker, Neilson, and Dowswell 2008; Parry et al. 2000.

23. Declercq et al. 2006.

24. Hofmeyr et al. 2009.

25. Hofmeyr, Gulmezoglu, and Pileggi 2010.

26. Zhang et al. 2010.

27. Clark et al. 2009a.

28. Alfirevic, Kelly, and Dowswell 2009.

29. Irion and Boulvain 2009; Mozurkewich et al. 2009.

30. Mozurkewich et al. 2009.

31. Declercq et al. 2006.

32. Ibid.

33. Fleischman, Oinuma, and Clark 2010.

34. Gulmezoglu, Crowther, and Middleton 2006.

35. Ibid., 2.

36. Davidoff et al. 2006.

37. Declercq et al. 2006.

38. Ibid.; Alfirevic, Kelly, and Dowswell 2009. For a discussion of choices of labor pain management available to women in the United States, see Marmor and Krol 2002. They find that women in the United States do not have options for pain relief available to women in advanced industrial democracies of western Europe.

39. Declercq et al. 2006.

40. Alfirevic, Kelly, and Dowswell 2009.

41. Ibid.

42. Anim-Somuah, Smyth, and Jones 2011.

43. Ibid.

44. Kotaska, Klein, and Liston 2006.

45. Anim-Somuah, Smyth, and Jones 2011.

46. Khunpradit, Lumbiganon, and Laopaiboon 2011; Declercq et al. 2006.

47. American College of Obstetricians and Gynecologists 2009.

48. Declercq et al. 2006; Albers and Krulewitch 1993.

49. American College of Obstetricians and Gynecologists 2009; Spencer et al. 1997; Nelson et al. 1996. According to Nelson and colleagues, in a population of 100,000 singleton children born at term, 2,324 would need to be delivered by c-section for an indication of a non-reassuring heart tone to prevent one child being born with cerebral palsy.

50. Grimes and Peipert 2010.

51. Alfirevic, Devane, and Gyte 2006.

52. American College of Obstetricians and Gynecologists 2009.

53. Declercq et al. 2006.

54. Ayres-de-Campos et al. 2011.

55. Morrison et al. 1993, 65.

56. Alfirevic, Devane, and Gyte 2006.

57. See, for example, Pettker and Lockwood 2008; Robinson 2008.

58. McNamara and Dildy 1999.

59. Spong et al. 2012.

60. Parer and Ikeda 2007.

61. Haas and Ayres 2002; Smith, Hernandez, and Wax 1997.

62. East, Begg, and Colditz 2010.

63. Arikan et al. 2000.

64. East, Begg, and Colditz 2010, 10.

65. Garite et al. 2000.

66. American College of Obstetricians and Gynecologists 2009.

67. Neilson 2012; Amer-Wahlin et al. 2011; Amer-Wahlin et al. 2001.

68. U.S. National Institutes of Health 2012.

69. Hofmeyr and Kulier 2012.

70. For a history of the use of forceps in childbirth, see Epstein 2010.

71. Spong et al. 2012.

72. Declercq et al. 2006.

Notes to Chapter 4

1. Declercq et al. 2006.

2. Martin et al. 2006.

3. Childbirth Connections 2012.

4. Gregory, Fridman, and Korst 2010.

5. Ibid.; Menacker, MacDorman, and Declercq 2010.

6. U.S. National Institutes of Health 1980.

7. Gregory, Fridman, and Korst 2010; Placek and Taffel 1988.

8. Grobman et al. 2011; Grobman 2010; Yeh et al. 2006.

9. Cragin 1916.

10. Gregory, Fridman, and Korst 2010; Wells 2010.

11. Discussed by Gregory, Fridman, and Korst 2010.

12. Noted by Wells 2010.

13. Ibid.

14. See Landon 2008 for a discussion of how accounts of uterine rupture began to flood medical journals.

15. McMahon et al. 1996; Wells 2010. In their 2010 *Seminars in Perinatology* article, Gregory, Fridman, and Korst discuss the effects of medical literature on VBAC rates. They make the point that the literature does not contain new findings on VBAC success rates or uterine rupture rates.

16. Gregory, Fridman, and Korst 2010.

17. Lydon-Rochelle et al. 2001; McMahon et al. 1996.

18. Public attention was also turned to an editorial by M. F. Greene (2001) that appeared in the same issue in which he questions the safety of VBAC.

19. Landon et al. 2004.

20. American College of Obstetricians and Gynecologists 2004; American College of Obstetricians and Gynecologists 1999.

21. Gregory, Fridman, and Korst 2010.

22. American College of Obstetricians and Gynecologists 1999.

23. Gregory, Fridman, and Korst 2010.

24. Mello 2001; Hyams et al. 1995.

25. Consensus Development Panel 2010.

26. Ibid.

27. American College of Obstetricians and Gynecologists 2010.

28. Ibid.

29. Ibid.

30. Ibid., 457.

31. Ibid.

32. Dodd et al. 2004.

33. Because no randomized controlled trials comparing VBAC and repeat c-section outcomes have been conducted, "current sources of information are limited to non-randomised cohort studies. Studies designed in this way have significant potential for bias and consequently conclusions based on these results are limited in their reliability and should be interpreted with caution" (ibid., 1).

34. Gregory, Fridman, and Korst 2010; McMahon et al. 1996. See also Lyerly et al. 2007 for a particularly poignant discussion about how values bear on decision making in pregnancy.

35. Oboro et al. 2010; Landon et al. 2004; McMahon et al. 1996.

36. Several studies have been unable to develop a predictive model of uterine rupture or maternal morbidity associated with VBAC attempts. These studies include Scifres et al. 2011; Eden et al. 2010; Grobman et al. 2008; Macones et al. 2006; McMahon et al. 1996.

37. Uterine rupture can also happen in women without a scarred uterus, but it is very uncommon. According to Zwart et al. 2009, the rate of uterine rupture is 5.1 per 10,000 women with a uterine scar and 0.8 per 10,000 women without a uterine scar.

38. The VBAC uterine rupture rate is reviewed in Landon 2008. The comparison of uterine rupture rates in VBAC attempts versus repeat c-sections is discussed by Macones et al. 2005; and Lydon-Rochelle et al. 2001.

39. Menacker, MacDorman, and Declercq 2010.

40. Consensus Development Panel 2010.

41. Guise et al. 2010.

42. Landon et al. 2004.

43. Menacker, MacDorman, and Declercq 2010.

44. O'Shea, Klebanoff, and Signore 2010.

45. Rozen, Ugoni, and Sheehan 2011.

46. Consensus Development Panel 2010; Smith et al. 2002.

47. See Roberts et al. 2007 for a discussion of this ethical argument.

48. Lin 2006.

49. Guise et al. 2010; Silver 2010.

50. Consensus Development Panel 2010.

51. Ibid.

52. Ibid.; Clark and Silver 2011; Silver 2010; Kuklina et al. 2009; Villar et al. 2007; Yang et al. 2007; Nisenblat et al. 2006; Dodd et al. 2004; Makoha et al. 2004.

53. Clark and Silver 2011; Silver 2010; Nisenblat et al. 2006.

54. Silver 2010; Flood et al. 2009.

55. Makoha et al. 2004, 231.

56. Gregory, Fridman, and Korst 2010.

57. Landon 2008; Roberts et al. 2007; Gochnour, Ratcliffe, and Stone 2005; Carr, Burkhardt, and Avery 2002.

58. Shihady et al. 2007. See also Perl 2010; Scott 2010; Paul 2009; Grady 2004.

59. International Cesarean Awareness Network 2012.

60. Ibid.

61. Shihady et al. 2007.
62. Klagholz and Strunk, 2012; Klagholz and Strunk 2009.
63. Ouzounian et al. 2011; Dekker et al. 2010; Landon 2010; Ogbonmwan et al. 2010; Weimar et al. 2010; Macones et al. 2006; Macones et al. 2005.
64. Scifres et al. 2011; Eden et al. 2010; Landon 2010; Grobman et al. 2008; Macones et al. 2006; Macones et al. 2005; McMahon et al. 1996.
65. Declercq et al. 2006.
66. Ibid.; Feldman et al. 2010; Cohen 2009.
67. Menacker, MacDorman, and Declercq 2010; Landon et al. 2004.
68. Rozen, Ugoni, and Sheehan 2011; Consensus Development Panel 2010; Smith et al. 2002.
69. Babbie 2010
70. Bujold 2010; Foureur et al. 2010.
71. Minkoff and Fridman 2010; Roberts et al. 2007.
72. Landon 2008; Roberts et al. 2007; Gochnour, Ratcliffe, and Stone 2005; Carr, Burkhardt, and Avery 2002.
73. Zinberg 2001, 568. Yang et al. 2009 find that malpractice premiums are linked to VBAC rates such that states with higher malpractice rates also have lower VBAC rates.
74. See Fineberg 2011 for the voice of a practicing obstetrician who is frustrated with the current constraints on practice she faces. See also Scott 2010; and Schneider 2005.
75. Sloan and Chepke 2008.
76. Ibid.
77. Leeman and King 2011, 127; Kuehn 2010.
78. Kuehn 2010, 1685.
79. Wells 2010.
80. Friedrich 1963.

Notes to Chapter 5

1. Kingdon et al. 2009; Annandale 1998.
2. Flavin 2009; Luna 2009; Smith 2005; Silliman et al. 2004.
3. Guttmacher Institute 2012.
4. See, for example, SisterSong Women of Color Reproductive Justice Collective 2012; Luna 2009; Smith 2005.
5. See Bender and de Gramont 2007 for an interesting book that explores the concept of choice across many different reproductive topics.
6. Declercq et al. 2006.

7. Feldman et al. 2010; Cohen 2009; Declercq et al. 2006.

8. Bernstein, Matalon-Grazi, and Rosenn 2012.

9. Ibid.

10. Ibid.

11. Ibid.

12. Caughey 2009, 251. Caughey contends that informed consent is presented in a way that suggests repeat c-section is without risk. See also Carr, Burkhardt, and Avery 2002, who suggest that midwives believe consent forms are designed to be scary to women.

13. Bernstein, Matalon-Grazi, and Barak Rosenn 2012; Goodall, McVittie, and Magill 2009; Moffat et al. 2007; Kamal et al. 2005.

14. Kamal et al. 2005.

15. Declercq et al. 2006.

16. Dunn and O'Herlihy 2005; Dodd, Pearce, and Crowther 2004.

17. MacDorman et al. 2008; Villar et al. 2007; Deneux-Tharaux et al. 2006.

18. Declercq et al. 2006.

19. Villar et al. 2007.

20. MacDorman et al. 2008.

21. A number of feminist scholars have examined the elevation of the status of the fetus over women in modern times. See, for example, Armstrong 2003; Roth 2000; Casper 1998; and Daniels 1993.

22. Declercq et al. 2006.

23. Ibid.

24. De Vries and De Vries 2007.

25. Declercq et al. 2006.

26. De Vries and De Vries 2007.

27. Declercq et al. 2006.

28. Lagan, Sinclair, and Kernohan 2010.

29. Song et al. 2012.

30. Morris and McInerney 2010.

31. Ibid. Also Elson 2009 shows that information in fictional television is very skewed.

32. Declercq et al. 2006.

33. American College of Obstetricians and Gynecologists 2008, 245.

34. Williams 2008.

35. Bernstein, Matalon-Grazi, and Rosenn 2012; Gamble and Creedy 2001.

36. Cyert and March 1963.

37. American Medical Association n.d. See Torres and De Vries 2009 for a cogent history of how the concept of ethics in health care developed over time.

38. Goldberg 2009; Torres and De Vries 2009; Rosenthal 2006.
39. Bergeron 2007, 481.
40. Habiba et al. 2006, 654.
41. Akkad et al. 2006; Akkad et al. 2004; Dixon-Woods et al. 2006.
42. Williams 2008. Nicette Jukelevics published what she considers an appropriate informed consent form for c-section, one that lists all risks of c-section, though this form is unlikely to be adopted by hospitals in the United States. See Jukelevics 2009.
43. Rosenthal 2006.
44. Christilaw 2006.
45. Goldberg 2009, 36.
46. Little et al. 2008; Leeman and Plante 2006.
47. Williams 2008.

Notes to the Conclusion

1. Clark et al. 2010.
2. Giddens 1971.
3. See Spong et al. 2012; and Sakala, Yang, and Corry 2013 for other ideas on how organizational changes can reduce the c-section rate and improve maternity care.
4. Declercq et al. 2006.
5. De Vries and De Vries 2007.
6. Spong et al. 2012.
7. Monari et al. 2008; Reime et al. 2004; Coco et al. 2000.
8. Little et al. 2012; Parry et al. 2000.
9. Irion and Boulvain 2009; Bricker, Neilson, and Dowswell 2008; Alsunnari et al. 2005; Sacks and Chen 2000; Ecker et al. 1997; Johnstone et al. 1996.
10. There are a number of studies that document these effects. See, for example, Simkin and O'Hara 2002; Kennell et al. 1991; Klaus et al. 1986. For a review that demonstrates the benefits of continuous support, see Hodnett et al. 2011.
11. Stapleton, Osborne, and Illuzzi 2013; Hutton, Reitsma, and Kaufman 2009.
12. Schroeder et al. 2012.
13. American Association of Birth Centers 2011.
14. MacDorman, Declercq, and Mathews 2011.
15. Mangesi, Hofmeyr, and Woods 2009.
16. Alfirevic, Devane, and Gyte 2006.
17. For a study on vaginal twin delivery, see Hofmeyr, Barrett, and Crowther

2011; for a study on vaginal breech delivery, see Hannah et al. 2004; and for a study on VBAC, see Dodd et al. 2004.

18. Declercq et al. 2006.

19. Scott 2010.

20. Hannah et al. 2000.

21. Simkin and O'Hara 2002; Kennell et al. 1991; Klaus et al. 1986. For a review that demonstrates the benefits of continuous support, see Hodnett et al. 2011.

22. Sakala, Yang, and Corry 2013.

23. Brennan, Sox, and Burstin 1996.

24. Gawande 2005. I am indebted to midwife Pam Grays for mentioning this solution and article to me.

25. Ibid.

26. This program does have its critics, who argue that the government is slow to compensate families and does not always recognize the disorders as being linked to vaccinations, even in the face of evidence. For a discussion of these critiques, see Levin 2004. However, just because there are critics of this program does not mean that it must be inefficient and ineffective.

27. For an example of ACOG's support, see American Congress of Obstetricians and Gynecologists, District II 2011.

28. See Siegal, Mello, and Studdert 2008.

29. Ibid.

30. Hamilton, Martin and Ventura 2012.

31. Siegal, Mello, and Studdert 2008.

32. This discussion is based on De Vries et al. 2009, in which they describe the model of Birth in the Netherlands and speculate on how other countries might adopt elements of the model.

33. Ibid.

34. Ibid.

35. World Health Organization 2012b.

36. De Vries et al. 2009.

37. Ibid.

38. American College of Obstetricians and Gynecologists 2011.

39. De Vries et al. 2009, 48.

40. World Health Organization 2012a.

41. In 2004 California established the California Maternal Quality Care Collaborative as a public health policy to examine maternal mortality. Other states should follow suit. Much information is available at California Maternity Quality Care Collaborative 2011.

42. Podulka, Stranges, and Steiner 2011.

43. Sakala, Delbanco, and Miller 2013.
44. Hamilton Martin, and Ventura 2012; Martin et al. 2012.
45. Zhani 2012.
46. Ibid.
47. Covert 2012.

Notes to the Methods Appendix

1. The author computed the percent of registered nurses who are women. Data available online at http://datawarehouse.hrsa.gov/nursingsurvey.aspx. The statistic on the percentage of female midwives comes from Sipe, Fullerton, and Schuiling 2009.
2. Calculations performed by the author. Data available from Smart 2012.
3. Smart 2012.
4. Calculations performed by the author. Data available from Smart 2012.
5. U.S. Department of Health and Human Services Health Resources and Services Administration 2010.
6. Sipe, Fullerton, and Schuiling 2009.

References

Abuhamad, Alfred, and ACOG Committee on Practice Bulletins—Obstetrics. 2008. ACOG practice bulletin, clinical management guidelines for obstetrician–gynecologists no. 98: Ultrasonography in pregnancy. *Obstetrics and Gynecology* 112 (4) (Oct): 951–61.

Abuhamad, Alfred, and William A. Grobman. 2010. Patient safety and medical liability: Current status and an agenda for the future. *Obstetrics and Gynecology* 116 (3) (Sep): 570–57.

Acker, David S., Benjamin P. Sachs, and Emanuel A. Friedman. 1985. Risk factors for shoulder dystocia. *Obstetrics and Gynecology* 66 (6) (Dec): 762–68.

Akkad, Andrea, Clare Jackson, Sara Kenyon, Mary Dixon-Woods, Nick Taub, and Marwan Habiba. 2006. Patients' perceptions of written consent: Questionnaire study. *BMJ (clinical research ed.)* 333 (7567) (Sep 9): 528.

———. 2004. Informed consent for elective and emergency surgery: Questionnaire study. *BJOG: An International Journal of Obstetrics and Gynaecology* 111 (10) (Oct): 1133–38.

Albers, Leah L., and Cara J. Krulewitch. 1993. Electronic fetal monitoring in the United States in the 1980s. *Obstetrics and Gynecology* 82 (1) (Jul): 8–10.

Alexander, James M., Kenneth J. Leveno, John Hauth, Mark B. Landon, Elizabeth Thom, Catherine Y. Spong, Michael W. Varner, Atef H. Moawad, Steve N. Caritis, Margaret Harper, Ronald J. Wapner, Yoram Sorokin, Menachem Miodovnik, Mary J. O'Sullivan, Baha M. Sibai, Oded Langer, and Steven G. Gabbe, for the National Institute of Child Health and Human Development Maternal-Fetal Medicine Units Network. 2006. Fetal injury associated with cesarean delivery. *Obstetrics and Gynecology* 108 (4) (Oct): 885–90.

Alfirevic, Zarko, Declan Devane, and Gillian M. L. Gyte. 2006. Continuous cardiotocography (CTG) as a form of electronic fetal monitoring (EFM) for fetal assessment during labour. *Cochrane Database of Systematic Reviews (online)* 3 (3) (Jul 19): CD006066.

Alfirevic, Zarko, Anthony J. Kelly, and Therese Dowswell. 2009. Intravenous oxytocin alone for cervical ripening and induction of labour. *Cochrane Database of Systematic Reviews (online)* 4 (4) (Oct 7): CD003246.

Alsunnari, Sahar, Howard Berger, Mathew Sermer, Gareth Seaward, Edmond Kelly, and Dan Farine. 2005. Obstetric outcome of extreme macrosomia. *Journal of Obstetrics and Gynaecology Canada* 27 (4) (Apr): 323–28.

American Association of Birth Centers. 2011. AABC press kit. Available from http://www.birthcenters.org/webfm_send/16 (accessed October 23, 2012).

American College of Obstetricians and Gynecologists. 2011. Committee opinion no. 476: Planned home birth. *Obstetrics and Gynecology* 117 (2, pt. 1) (Feb): 425–28.

———. 2010. ACOG practice bulletin no. 115: Vaginal birth after previous cesarean delivery. *Obstetrics and Gynecology* 116 (2, pt. 1) (Aug): 450–63.

———. 2009. ACOG practice bulletin no. 106: Intrapartum fetal heart rate monitoring: Nomenclature, interpretation, and general management principles. *Obstetrics and Gynecology* 114 (1) (Jul): 192–202.

———. 2008. ACOG committee opinion no. 395. Surgery and patient choice. *Obstetrics and Gynecology* 111 (1) (Jan): 243–47.

———. 2006. ACOG committee opinion no. 340: Mode of term singleton breech delivery. *Obstetrics and Gynecology* 108 (1) (Jul): 235–37.

———. 2004. ACOG practice bulletin no. 54: Vaginal birth after previous cesarean. *Obstetrics and Gynecology* 104 (1) (Jul): 203–12.

———. 1999. ACOG practice bulletin no. 5: Vaginal birth after previous cesarean delivery. *International Journal of Gynaecology and Obstetrics: The Official Organ of the International Federation of Gynaecology and Obstetrics* 66 (2) (Aug): 197–204.

American Congress of Obstetricians and Gynecologists, District II. 2011. S2445 Hannon No Assembly Companion. Available from http://www.acog.org/About_ACOG/ACOG_Districts/District_II/S_2445__Hannon____No_Assembly_Companion (accessed on February 18, 2013).

American Medical Association. n.d. Informed consent. Available from http://www.ama-assn.org/ama/pub/physician-resources/legal-topics/patient-physician-relationship-topics/informed-consent.page (accessed on October 13, 2012).

Amer-Wahlin, Isis, Charlotte Hellsten, Håkan Norén, Henrik Hagberg, Andreas Herbst, Ingemar Kjellmer, Håkan Lilja, Claes Lindoff, Maivi Månsson, Laila Mårtensson, Per Olofsson, Anna-Karin Sundström, and Karel Marsál. 2001. Cardiotocography only versus cardiotocography plus ST analysis of fetal electrocardiogram for intrapartum fetal monitoring: A Swedish randomised controlled trial. *Lancet* 358 (9281) (Aug 18): 534–38.

Amer-Wahlin, Isis, Ingemar Kjellmer, Karel Marsal, Per Olofsson, and Karl Gustaf Rosen. 2011. Swedish randomized controlled trial of cardiotocography only versus cardiotocography plus ST analysis of fetal electrocardiogram revisited: Analysis of data according to standard versus modified intention-to-treat principle. *Acta Obstetricia et Gynecologica Scandinavica* 90 (9) (Sep): 990–96.

Anderson, Gerard F., Peter S. Hussey, Bianca K. Frogner, and Hugh R. Waters. 2005. Health spending in the United States and the rest of the industrialized world. *Health Affairs* 24 (4): 903–14.

Anderson, Jenny. 2012. Private schools mine parents' data, and wallets. *New York Times*. March 26.

Anim-Somuah, Millicent, Rebecca Smyth, and Leanne Jones. 2011. Epidural versus non-epidural or no analgesia in labour. *Cochrane Database of Systematic Reviews (online)* 12 (12) (Dec 7): CD000331.

Annandale, Ellen. 1998. *The sociology of health and medicine: A critical introduction.* Cambridge, UK: Polity Press.

Arikan, Gürkan M., Heinz S. Scholz, Martin C. Haeusler, Albrecht Giuliani, Josef Haas, and Peter A. M. Weiss. 2000. Low fetal oxygen saturation at birth and acidosis. *Obstetrics and Gynecology* 95 (4) (Apr): 565–71.

Armstrong, Elizabeth M. 2003. *Conceiving risk, bearing responsibility: Fetal alcohol syndrome and the diagnosis of moral disorder.* Baltimore: Johns Hopkins University Press.

Aron, David C., Howard S. Gordon, David L. DiGiuseppe, Dwain L. Harper, and Gary E. Rosenthal. 2000. Variations in risk-adjusted cesarean delivery rates according to race and health insurance. *Medical Care* 38 (1) (Jan): 35–44.

Ayres-de-Campos, D., D. Arteiro, C. Costa-Santos, and J. Bernardes. 2011. Knowledge of adverse neonatal outcome alters clinicians' interpretation of the intrapartum cardiotocography. *BJOG: An International Journal of Obstetrics and Gynaecology* 118 (8) (Jul): 978–84.

Babbie, Earl. 2010. *The practice of social research.* Belmont, CA: Wadsworth.

Baker, Tom. 2005. *Medical malpractice myth.* Chicago: University of Chicago Press.

Baldwin, Laura-Mae, Gary Hart, Michael Lloyd, Meredith Fordyce, and Roger A. Rosenblatt. 1995. Defensive medicine and obstetrics. *JAMA: The Journal of the American Medical Association* 274 (2) (Nov 22–29): 1606–10.

Bender, Karen E., and Nina de Gramont. 2007. *Choice: True stories of birth, contraception, infertility, adoption, single parenthood, and abortion.* San Francisco: MacAdam/Cage.

Benedetti, Thomas J., Laura-Mae Baldwin, Susan M. Skillman, C. Holly A. Andrilla, Elise Bowditch, Katherine Camacho Carr, and Susan J. Myers. 2006.

Professional liability issues and practice patterns of obstetric providers in Washington State. *Obstetrics and Gynecology* 107 (6) (Jun): 1238–46.

Ben-Haroush, Avi, Yariv Yogev, Jacob Bar, Hagit Glickman, Boris Kaplan, and Moshe Hod. 2004. Indicated labor induction with vaginal prostaglandin E2 increases the risk of cesarean section even in multiparous women with no previous cesarean section. *Journal of Perinatal Medicine* 32 (1): 31–36.

Benson, J. Kenneth. 1977. Organizations: A dialectical view. *Administrative Science Quarterly* 22 (1) (Mar): 1–21.

Bergeron, Veronique. 2007. The ethics of cesarean section on maternal request: A feminist critique of the American college of obstetricians and gynecologists' position on patient-choice surgery. *Bioethics* 21 (9) (Nov): 478–87.

Bernstein, Sarah N., Shira Matalon-Grazi, and Barak M. Rosenn. 2012. Trial of labor versus repeat cesarean: Are patients making an informed decision? *American Journal of Obstetrics and Gynecology* 207 (Sep): 204.e1–e6.

Blair, Eve, and Fiona Stanley. 1993. When can cerebral palsy be prevented? The generation of causal hypotheses by multivariate analysis of a case-control study. *Paediatric and Perinatal Epidemiology* 7 (3) (Jul): 272–301.

Boston Women's Health Book Collective. 2008. *Our bodies, ourselves: Pregnancy and birth*. New York: Simon & Schuster.

Boyle, Elaine M., Gary Poulsen, David J. Field, Jennifer J. Kurinczuk, Dieter Wolke, Zarko Alfirevic, and Maria A. Quigley. 2012. Effects of gestational age at birth on health outcomes at 3 and 5 years of age: Population-based cohort study. *BMJ (online)* 344 (Mar).

Brennan, Troyen A., Colin M. Sox, and Helen R. Burstin. 1996. Relation between negligent adverse events and the outcomes of medical-malpractice litigation. *New England Journal of Medicine* 335 (26) (Dec 26): 1963–67.

Bricker, Leanne, James P. Neilson, and Therese Dowswell. 2008. Routine ultrasound in late pregnancy (after 24 weeks gestation). *Cochrane Database of Systematic Reviews (online)* 4 (4) (Oct 8): CD001451.

Brown, H. Shelton, III. 2007. Lawsuit activity, defensive medicine, and small area variation: The case of cesarean sections revisited. *Health Economics, Policy, and Law* 2 (3) (Jul): 285–96.

Bujold, Emmanuel. 2010. Evaluating professional society guidelines on vaginal birth after cesarean. *Seminars in Perinatology* 34 (5) (Oct): 314–17.

California Maternity Quality Care Collaborative. 2011. *California Pregnancy-Associated Mortality Review*. Available from http://www.cdph.ca.gov/data/statistics/Pages/CaliforniaPregnancy-AssociatedMortalityReview.aspx (accessed January 29, 2013).

Callaghan, William M., Andreea A. Creanga, and Elena V. Kuklina. 2012. Severe maternal morbidity among delivery and postpartum hospitalizations in the United States. *Obstetrics and Gynecology* 120 (5) (Nov): 1029–36.

Carr, Catherine A., Patricia Burkhardt, and Melissa Avery. 2002. Vaginal birth after cesarean birth: A national survey of U.S. midwifery practice. *Journal of Midwifery and Women's Health* 47 (5) (Sep/Oct): 347–52.

Casper, Monica J. 1998. *The making of the unborn patient*. New Brunswick: Rutgers University Press.

Catlin, Aaron, Cathy Cowan, Micah Hartman, Stephen Heffler, and the National Health Expenditure Accounts Team. 2008. National health spending in 2006. *Health Affairs (Project Hope)* 27 (1) (2008): 1–16.

Caughey, Aaron B. 2009. Informed consent for a vaginal birth after previous cesarean delivery. *Journal of Midwifery and Women's Health* 54 (3) (May/Jun): 249–53.

Center for Studying Health System Change. 2008. Health Tracking Physician Survey, 2008 [United States]. ICPSR27202-v1. Ann Arbor, MI: Inter-university Consortium for Political and Social Research [distributor], 2010-02-16. doi:10.3886/ICPSR27202.v1.

Centers for Disease Control and Prevention. 2012. Infant, neonatal, and maternal mortality rates by race. Available from http://www.census.gov/compendia/statab/cats/births_deaths_marriages_divorces.html (accessed March 5, 2012).

———. 1995. Rates of cesarean delivery: United States, 1993. *Morbidity and Mortality Weekly Report* 44 (15) (Apr 21): 303–7.

Centner, Terence J. 2008. *America's blame culture: Pointing fingers and shunning restitution*. Durham, NC: Carolina Academic Press.

Childbirth Connections. 2012. Rates for total cesarean section, primary cesarean section, and vaginal birth after cesarean (VBAC), United States, 1989–2010. Available from http://www.childbirthconnection.org/article.asp?ck=10554 (accessed September 18, 2012).

Christilaw, Jan E. 2006. Cesarean section by choice: Constructing a reproductive rights framework for the debate. *International Journal of Gynaecology and Obstetrics: The Official Organ of the International Federation of Gynaecology and Obstetrics* 94 (3) (Sep): 262–68.

Clark, Erin A. S., and Robert Silver. 2011. Long-term maternal morbidity associated with repeat cesarean delivery. *American Journal of Obstetrics and Gynecology* 205 (6 Supplement) (Dec): S2–10.

Clark, Steven L., Michael A. Belfort, Spencer L. Byrum, Janet A. Meyers, and Jonathan B. Perlin. 2008a. Improved outcomes, fewer cesarean deliveries, and reduced litigation: Results of a new paradigm in patient safety. *American Journal of Obstetrics and Gynecology* 199 (2) (Aug): 105.e1–e7.

Clark, Steven L., Michael A. Belfort, Gary A. Dildy, and Janet A. Meyers. 2008b. Reducing obstetric litigation through alterations in practice patterns. *Obstetrics and Gynecology* 112 (6) (Dec): 1279–83.

Clark, Steven L., Donna R. Frye, Janet A. Meyers, Michael A. Belfort, Gary A. Dildy, Shalece Kofford, Jane Englebright, and Jonathan A. Perlin. 2010. Reduction in elective delivery at <39 weeks of gestation: Comparative effectiveness of 3 approaches to change and the impact on neonatal intensive care admission and stillbirth. *American Journal of Obstetrics and Gynecology* 203 (5) (Nov): 449.e1–e6.

Clark, Steven L., and Gary D. Hankins. 2003. Temporal and demographic trends in cerebral palsy: Fact and fiction. *American Journal of Obstetrics and Gynecology* 188 (3) (Mar): 628–33.

Clark, Steven L., Janet A. Meyers, Donna K. Frye, and Jonathan A. Perlin. 2011. Patient safety in obstetrics: The hospital corporation of America experience. *American Journal of Obstetrics and Gynecology* 204 (4) (Apr): 283–87.

Clark, Steven L., Darla D. Miller, Michael A. Belfort, Gary A. Dildy, Donna K. Frye, and Janet A. Meyers. 2009a. Neonatal and maternal outcomes associated with elective-term delivery. *American Journal of Obstetrics and Gynecology* 200 (2) (Feb): 156.e1–e4.

Clark, Steven L., Kathleen Rice Simpson, G. Eric Knox, and Thomas J. Garite. 2009b. Oxytocin: New perspectives on an old drug. *American Journal of Obstetrics and Gynecology* 200 (1) (Jan): 35.e1–e6.

Coco, Andrew S., Thomas J. Gates, Mary E. Gallagher, and Michael A. Horst. 2000. Association of attending physician specialty with the cesarean delivery rate in the same patient population. *Clinical Research and Methods* 32 (9): 639–44.

Cohen, Elizabeth. 2009. Mom fights, gets the delivery she wants. *CNN Health.* December 17. Available from http://articles.cnn.com/ (accessed September 18, 2011).

Collins, Randall. 1986. *Max Weber: A skeleton key.* Masters of social theory no. 3. Beverly Hills: Sage.

Consensus Development Panel. 2010. National Institutes of Health consensus development conference statement: Vaginal birth after cesarean: New insights. *Obstetrics and Gynecology* 115 (6) (June): 1279–95.

Covert, Bryce. 2012. Why the Obamacare decision is very good news for women. *Forbes.* June 28. Available at http://www.forbes.com/sites/brycecovert/2012/06/28/obamacare-decision-why-women-are-the-big-winners-health-care-supreme-court/ (accessed October 22, 2012).

Cragin, Edwin B. 1916. Conservatism in obstetrics. *New York Medical Journal* 104 (1) (July): 1–3.

Cyert, Richard Michael, and James G. March. 1963. *Behavioral theory of the firm*. Prentice-Hall international series in management; Prentice-Hall behavioral sciences in business series. Englewood Cliffs, NJ: Prentice-Hall.

Daltveit, Anne Kjersti, Mette Christophersen Tollånes, Hege Pihlstrøm, and Lorentz M. Irgens. 2008. Cesarean delivery and subsequent pregnancies. *Obstetrics and Gynecology* 111 (6) (Jun): 1327–34.

Daniels, Cynthia R. 1993. *At Women's Expense: State Power and the Politics of Fetal Rights*. Cambridge: Harvard University Press.

Davidoff, Michael J., Todd Dias, Karla Damus, Rebecca Russell, Vani R. Bettegowda, Siobhan Dolan, Richard H. Schwarz, Nancy S. Green, and Joann Petrini. 2006. Changes in the gestational age distribution among U.S. singleton births: Impact on rates of late preterm birth, 1992 to 2002. *Seminars in Perinatology* 30 (1) (Feb): 8–15.

Davis-Floyd, Robbie. 1992. *Birth as an American rite of passage*. Comparative studies of health systems and medical care no. 35. Berkeley: University of California Press.

Davis-Floyd, Robbie, and Carolyn Fishel Sargent, eds. 1997. *Childbirth and authoritative knowledge: Cross-cultural perspectives*. Berkeley: University of California Press.

De Vries, Charlotte A., and Raymond G. De Vries. 2007. Childbirth education in the 21st century: An immodest proposal. *Journal of Perinatal Education* 16 (4) (Fall): 38–48.

De Vries, Raymond, Therese A. Wiegers, Beatrijs Smulders, and Edwin van Teijlingen. 2009. The Dutch obstetrical system: Vanguard of the future in maternity care. Pp. 31–53 in *Birth Models That Work*, edited by Robbie Davis-Floyd, Lesley Barclay, Betty-Anne Daviss, and Jan Tritten. Berkeley: University of California Press.

Declercq, Eugene, Mary Barger, Howard J. Cabral, Stephen R. Evans, Milton Kotelchuck, Carol Simon, Judith Weiss, and Linda J. Heffner. 2007. Maternal outcomes associated with planned primary cesarean births compared with planned vaginal births. *Obstetrics and Gynecology* 109 (3) (Mar): 669–77.

Declercq, Eugene, Deborah K. Cunningham, Cynthia Johnson, and Carol Sakala. 2008. Mothers' reports of postpartum pain associated with vaginal and cesarean deliveries: Results of a national survey. *Birth (Berkeley, CA)* 35 (1) (Mar): 16–24.

Declercq, Eugene, Fay Menacker, and Marian MacDorman. 2005. Rise in "no indicated risk" primary caesareans in the United States, 1991–2001: Cross sectional analysis. *BMJ (clinical research ed.)* 330 (7482) (Jan 8): 71–72.

Declercq, Eugene, Carol Sakala, Maureen Corry, and Sandra Applebaum. 2006. *Listening to mothers II: Report of the second national U.S. survey of women's childbearing experiences.* Childbirth Connection. Available from http://www.childbirthconnection.org/article.asp?ck=10401 (accessed September 14, 2011).

Dekker, G. A., A. Chan, C. G. Luke, K. Priest, M. Riley, J. Halliday, J. F. King, V. Gee, M. O'Neill, M. Snell, V. Cull, and S. Cornes. 2010. Risk of uterine rupture in Australian women attempting vaginal birth after one prior caesarean section: A retrospective population-based cohort study. *BJOG An International Journal of Obstetrics and Gynaecology* 117 (11) (Oct): 1358–65.

Dekker, Rebecca. 2012. What is the evidence for using an external cephalic version to turn a breech baby? Available at http://evidencebasedbirth.com/what-is-the-evidence-for-using-an-external-cephalic-version-to-turn-a-breech-baby/ (accessed October 23, 2012).

Deneux-Tharaux, Catherine, Elodie Carmona, Marie-Hélene Bouvier-Colle, and Gérard Bréart. 2006. Postpartum maternal mortality and cesarean delivery. *Obstetrics and Gynecology* 108 (3, pt. 1) (Sep): 541–48.

Devane, Declan, Joan G. Lalor, Sean Daly, William McGuire, and Valerie Smith. 2012. Cardiotocography versus intermittent auscultation of fetal heart on admission to labour ward for assessment of fetal well-being. *Cochrane Database of Systematic Reviews (online)* 2 (2) (Feb 15): CD005122.

Dixon-Woods, Mary, Simon J. Williams, Clare J. Jackson, Andrea Akkad, Sara Kenyon, and Marwan Habiba. 2006. Why do women consent to surgery, even when they do not want to? An interactionist and Bourdieusian analysis. *Social Science and Medicine* 62 (11) (June): 2742–53.

Dodd, Jodie M., Caroline A. Crowther, Erasmo Huertas, Jeanne-Marie Guise, and Dell Horey. 2004. Planned elective repeat caesarean section versus planned vaginal birth for women with a previous caesarean birth. *Cochrane Database of Systematic Reviews (online)* 4 (4) (Oct 18): CD004224.

Dodd, Jodie, Elizabeth Pearce, and Caroline Crowther. 2004. Women's experiences and preferences following caesarean birth. *Australian and New Zealand Journal of Obstetrics and Gynaecology* 44 (6) (Dec): 521–24.

Dranove, David, and Yasutora Watanabe. 2010. Influence and deterrence: How obstetricians respond to litigation against themselves and their colleagues. *American Law and Economics Review* 12 (1) (March 20): 69–94.

Dubay, Lisa, Robert Kaestner, and Timothy Waidmann. 1999. The impact of malpractice fears on cesarean section rates. *Journal of Health Economics* 18 (4) (Aug): 491–522.

Dumont, Alexandre, Luc de Bernis, Marie-Hélène. H. Bouvier-Colle, and Gérard Bréart for the MOMA Study Group. 2001. Caesarean section rate for maternal indication in sub-Saharan Africa: A systematic review. *Lancet* 358 (9290) (Oct 20): 1328–33.

Dunn, Elizabeth A., and Colm O'Herlihy. 2005. Comparison of maternal satisfaction following vaginal delivery after caesarean section and caesarean section after previous vaginal delivery. *European Journal of Obstetrics, Gynecology, and Reproductive Biology* 121 (1) (Jul 1): 56–60.

East, Christine E., Lisa Begg, and Paul B. Colditz. 2010. Fetal pulse oximetry for fetal assessment in labour. *Cochrane Database of Systematic Reviews (online)* 2 (2) (Feb 17): CD004075.

Ecker, Jeffrey L., James A. Greenberg, Errol R. Norwitz, Allan S. Nadel, and John T. Repke. 1997. Birth weight as a predictor of brachial plexus injury. *Obstetrics and Gynecology* 89 (5, pt. 1) (May): 643–47.

Eden, Karen B., Marian McDonagh, Mary Anna Denman, Nicole Marshall, Cathy Emeis, Rongwei Fu, Rosalind Janik, Miranda Walker, and Jeanne-Marie Guise. 2010. New insights on vaginal birth after cesarean: Can it be predicted? *Obstetrics and Gynecology* 116 (4) (Oct): 967–81.

Ekstrom, Asa, Daniel Altman, Ingela Wiklund, Christina Larsson, and Ellika Andolf. 2008. Planned cesarean section versus planned vaginal delivery: Comparison of lower urinary tract symptoms. *International Urogynecology Journal and Pelvic Floor Dysfunction* 19 (4) (Apr): 459–65.

Elson, Vicki. 2009. *Laboring under an illusion.* DVD. Available from http://birth-media.com/.

Epstein, Randi Hutton. 2010. *Get me out: A history of childbirth from the Garden of Eden to the sperm bank.* New York: Norton.

Faundes, A., T. Guarisi, and A. M. Pinto-Neto. 2001. The risk of urinary incontinence of parous women who delivered only by cesarean section. *International Journal of Gynaecology and Obstetrics: The Official Organ of the International Federation of Gynaecology and Obstetrics* 72 (1) (Jan): 41–46.

Fawole, Bukola, and G. Justus Hofmeyr. 2012. Maternal oxygen administration for fetal distress. *Cochrane Database of Systematic Reviews (online)* 12 (12) (Dec 12): CD000136.

Feldman, Perle, Rivka Cymbalist, Saraswathi Vedam, and Andrew Kotaska. 2010. Roundtable discussion: "No one can condemn you to a C-section!" *Birth (Berkeley, CA)* 37 (3) (Sep): 245–51.

Fineberg, Annette E. 2011. An obstetrician's lament. *Obstetrics and Gynecology* 117 (5) (May): 1188–90.

Flavin, Jeanne. 2009. *Our bodies, our crimes: The policing of women's reproduction in America.* Alternative criminology series. New York: New York University Press.

Fleischman, Alan R., Motoko Oinuma, and Steven L. Clark. 2010. Rethinking the definition of "term pregnancy." *Obstetrics and Gynecology* 116 (1) (Jul): 136–39.

Flood, Karen M., Soha Said, Michael Geary, Michael Robson, Christopher Fitzpatrick, and Fergal D. Malone. 2009. Changing trends in peripartum hysterectomy over the last 4 decades. *American Journal of Obstetrics and Gynecology* 200 (6) (Jun): 632.e1–e6.

Foad, Susan L., Charles T. Mehlman, and Jun Ying. 2008. The Epidemiology of Neonatal Brachial Plexus Palsy in the United States. *Journal of Bone and Joint Surgery* 90 (6): 1258–64.

Foureur, Maralyn, Clare L. Ryan, Michael Nicholl, and Caroline Homer. 2010. Inconsistent evidence: Analysis of six national guidelines for vaginal birth after cesarean section. *Birth (Berkeley, CA)* 37 (1) (Mar): 3–10.

Friedrich, Carl J. 1963. *Man and his government: An empirical theory of politics.* New York: McGraw-Hill.

Fritel, Xavier, Virginie Ringa, Noelle Varnoux, Arnaud Fauconnier, Stephanie Piault, and Gerard Breart. 2005. Mode of delivery and severe stress incontinence: A cross-sectional study among 2,625 perimenopausal women. *BJOG: An International Journal of Obstetrics and Gynaecology* 112 (12) (Dec): 1646–51.

Fuchs, Karin, and Cynthia Gyamfi. 2008. The influence of obstetric practices on late prematurity. *Clinics in Perinatology* 35 (2) (Jun): 343–60.

Gamble, Jenny A., and Debra K. Creedy. 2001. Women's preference for a cesarean section: Incidence and associated factors. *Birth (Berkeley, CA)* 28 (2) (Jun): 101–10.

———. 2000. Women's request for a cesarean section: A critique of the literature. *Birth (Berkeley, CA)* 27 (4) (Dec): 256–63.

Garite, Thomas J., Gary A. Dildy, Helen McNamara, Michael P. Nageotte, Frank H. Boehm, Eric H. Dellinger, Robert A. Knuppel, Richard P. Porreco, Hugh S. Miller, Shiraz Sunderji, Michael W. Varner, and David B. Swedlow. 2000. A multicenter controlled trial of fetal pulse oximetry in the intrapartum management of nonreassuring fetal heart rate patterns. *American Journal of Obstetrics and Gynecology* 183 (5) (Nov): 1049–58.

Gawande, Atul. 2006. The score: How childbirth went industrial. *New Yorker.* October 9.

———. 2005. The malpractice mess: Who pays the price when patients sue doctors? *New Yorker.* November 14.

GE Healthcare. 1997. Electronic fetal heart rate monitoring: Research guidelines for interpretation. *American Journal of Obstetrics and Gynecology* 177 (6): 1385–90.

Gherman, Robert B., Suneet Chauhan, Joseph G. Ouzounian, Henry Lerner, Bernard Gonik, and T. Murphy Goodwin. 2006. Shoulder dystocia: The unpreventable obstetric emergency with empiric management guidelines. *American Journal of Obstetrics and Gynecology* 195 (3) (Sep): 657–72.

Giddens, Anthony. 1971. *Capitalism and modern social theory: An analysis of the writings of Marx, Durkheim, and Max Weber.* Cambridge: Cambridge University Press.

Gillum, Jack, and Marisol Bello. 2011. When standardized test scores soared in DC, were the gains real? *USA Today*, March 27, 2011.

Ginsburg, Faye D., and Rayna Rapp. 1995. *Conceiving the new world order: The global politics of reproduction.* Berkeley: University of California Press.

Glantz, J. Christopher. 2011. Rates of labor induction and primary cesarean delivery do not correlate with rates of adverse neonatal outcome in level I hospitals. *Journal of Maternal–Fetal and Neonatal Medicine: The Official Journal of the European Association of Perinatal Medicine, the Federation of Asia and Oceania Perinatal Societies, the International Society of Perinatal Obstetricians* 24 (4) (Apr): 636–42.

Glazener, C. M., G. P. Herbison, C. MacArthur, R. Lancashire, M. A. McGee, A. M. Grant, and P. D. Wilson. 2006. New postnatal urinary incontinence: Obstetric and other risk factors in primiparae. *BJOG: An International Journal of Obstetrics and Gynaecology* 113 (2) (Feb): 208–17.

Glezerman, Marek. 2006. Five years to the term breech trial: The rise and fall of a randomized controlled trial. *American Journal of Obstetrics and Gynecology* 194 (1) (Jan): 20–25.

Gochnour, Greg, Stephen Ratcliffe, and Mary Bishop Stone. 2005. The Utah VBAC study. *Maternal and Child Health Journal* 9 (2) (Jun): 181–88.

Goldberg, Holly. 2009. Informed decision making in maternity care. *Journal of Perinatal Education* 18 (1): 32–40.

Goodall, Karen Elizabeth, Chris McVittie, and Michelle Magill. 2009. Birth choice following primary caesarean section: Mothers' perceptions of the influence of health professionals on decision making. *Journal of Reproductive and Infant Psychology* 27 (1): 4–14.

Goodrick, Elizabeth, and Gerald R. Salancik. 1996. Organizational discretion in responding to institutional practices: Hospitals and cesarean births. *Administrative Science Quarterly* 41 (1) (Mar): 1 28.

Gossman, Ginger L., Jutta M. Joesch, and Koray Tanfer. 2006. Trends in maternal request cesarean delivery from 1991 to 2004. *Obstetrics and Gynecology* 108 (6) (Dec): 1506–16.

Grady, Denise. 2008. After cesareans, some see higher insurance costs. *New York Times.* June 1.

———. 2004. Repeat cesareans becoming harder to avoid. *New York Times.* November 29.

Grant, Darren, and Melayne Morgan McInnes. 2004. Malpractice experience and the incidence of cesarean delivery: A physician-level longitudinal analysis. *Inquiry: A Journal of Medical Care Organization, Provision, and Financing* 41 (2) (Summer): 170–88.

Gray, R., M. A. Quigley, C. Hockley, J. J. Kurinczuk, M. Goldacre, and P. Brocklehurst. 2007. Caesarean delivery and risk of stillbirth in subsequent pregnancy: A retrospective cohort study in an English population. *BJOG: An International Journal of Obstetrics and Gynaecology* 114 (3) (Mar): 264–70.

Greenberg, Michael D., Amelia M. Haviland, J. Scott Ashwood, and Regan Main. 2010. *Is better patient safety associated with less malpractice activity? Evidence from California.* Technical reports. Santa Monica, CA: RAND Corporation.

Greene, Michael F. 2001. Vaginal delivery after cesarean section: Is the risk acceptable? *New England Journal of Medicine* 345 (1) (Jul 5): 54–55.

Gregory, Kimberly D., Moshe Fridman, and Lisa Korst. 2010. Trends and patterns of vaginal birth after cesarean availability in the United States. *Seminars in Perinatology* 34 (4) (Aug): 237–43.

Greve, Paul. 2009. Labor pains: Liability trends in obstetrics. *Medical Liability Monitor* 34 (8): 4–5, 7.

Grimes, David A., and Jeffrey F. Peipert. 2010. Electronic fetal monitoring as a public health screening program: The arithmetic of failure. *Obstetrics and Gynecology* 116 (6) (Dec): 1397–1400.

Grobman, William A. 2010. Rates and prediction of successful vaginal birth after cesarean. *Seminars in Perinatology* 34 (4) (Aug): 244–48.

Grobman, William A., Yinglei Lai, Mark B. Landon, Catherine Y. Spong, Kenneth J. Leveno, Dwight J. Rouse, Michael W. Varner, Atef H. Moawad, Steve N. Caritis, Margaret Harper, Ronald J. Wapner, Yoram Sorokin, Menachem Miodovnik, Marshall Carpenter, Mary J. O'Sullivan, Baha M. Sibai, Oded Langer, John M. Thorp, Susan M. Ramin, and Brian M. Mercer. 2008. Prediction of uterine rupture associated with attempted vaginal birth after cesarean delivery. *American Journal of Obstetrics and Gynecology* 199 (1) (Jul): 30.e1–e5.

Grobman, William A., Yinglei Lai, Mark B. Landon, Catherine Y. Spong, Dwight J. Rouse, Michael W. Varner, Steve N. Caritis, Margaret Harper, Ronald J. Wapner, and Yoram Sorokin. 2011. The change in the rate of vaginal birth after caesarean section. *Paediatric and Perinatal Epidemiology* 25 (1) (Jan): 37–43.

Guise, Jeanne-Marie, Mary Anna Denman, Cathy Emeis, Nicole Marshall, Miranda Walker, Rongwei Fu, Rosalind Janik, Peggy Nygren, Karen B. Eden, and Marian McDonagh. 2010. Vaginal birth after cesarean: New insights on maternal and neonatal outcomes. *Obstetrics and Gynecology* 115 (6): 1267–78.

Gulmezoglu, A. Metin, Caroline A. Crowther, and Philippa Middleton. 2006. Induction of labour for improving birth outcomes for women at or beyond term. *Cochrane Database of Systematic Reviews (online)* 4 (4) (Oct 18): CD004945.

Guttmacher Institute. 2012. State policies in brief: Requirements for ultrasound. Available from http://www.guttmacher.org/statecenter/spibs/index.html (accessed October 5, 2012).

Haas, David M., and Allen W. Ayres. 2002. Laceration injury at cesarean section. *Journal of Maternal–Fetal and Neonatal Medicine: The Official Journal of the European Association of Perinatal Medicine, the Federation of Asia and Oceania Perinatal Societies, the International Society of Perinatal Obstetricians* 11 (3) (Mar): 196–98.

Habiba, M., M. Kaminski, M. Da Fre, K. Marsal, O. Bleker, J. Librero, H. Grandjean, P. Gratia, S. Guaschino, W. Heyl, D. Taylor, and M. Cuttini. 2006. Caesarean section on request: A comparison of obstetricians' attitudes in eight European countries. *BJOG: An International Journal of Obstetrics and Gynaecology* 113 (6) (Jun): 647–56.

Halpern, Stephen H., Barbara L. Leighton, Arne Ohlsson, John F. R. Barrett, and Amy Rice. 1998. Effect of epidural versus parenteral opioid analgesia on the progress of labor. *Journal of the American Medical Association* 80 (24): 2105–10.

Hamilton, Brady E., Joyce A. Martin, and Stephanie J. Ventura. 2012. Births: Preliminary data for 2011. *National Vital Statistics Report* 61 (5): 1–19.

Hannah, Mary E., Walter J. Hannah, Sheila A. Hewson, Ellen D. Hodnett, Saroj Saigal, and Andrew R. Willan. 2000. Planned caesarean section versus planned vaginal birth for breech presentation at term: A randomised multicentre trial. Term breech trial collaborative group. *Lancet* 356 (9239) (Oct 21): 1375–83.

Hannah, Mary E., Hilary Whyte, Walter J. Hannah, Sheila Hewson, Kofi Amankwah, Mary Cheng, Amiram Gafni, Patricia Guselle, Michael Helewa, Ellen D. Hodnett, Eileen Hutton, Rose Kung, Darren McKay, Susan Ross, Saroj Saigal, Andrew Willan, and the Term Breech Trial Collaborative Group. 2004. Maternal outcomes at 2 years after planned cesarean section versus planned vaginal birth for breech presentation at term: The international randomized term breech trial. *American Journal of Obstetrics and Gynecology* 191 (3) (Sep): 917–27.

Hansen, Anne Kirkeby, Kirsten Wisborg, Niels Uldbjerg, and Tine Brink Henriksen. 2008. Risk of respiratory morbidity in term infants delivered by elective caesarean section: Cohort study. *BMJ (clinical research ed.)* 336 (7635) (Jan 12): 85–87.

Hay, Iain. 1992. *Money, medicine, and malpractice in American society.* New York: Praeger.

Hendrix, Nancy W., Suneet P. Chauhan, James A. Scardo, Janna M. Ellings, and Lawrence D. Devoe. 2000. Managing nonreassuring fetal heart rate patterns before cesarean delivery: Compliance with ACOG recommendations. *Journal of Reproductive Medicine* 45 (12) (Dec): 995–99.

Hendrix, Susan L., Amanda Clark, Ingrid Nygaard, Aaron Aragaki, Vanessa Barnabei, and Anne McTiernan. 2002. Pelvic organ prolapse in the women's health initiative: Gravity and gravidity. *American Journal of Obstetrics and Gynecology* 186 (6) (Jun): 1160–66.

Hodnett, Ellen D., Simon Gates, G. Justus Hofmeyr, Carol Sakala, and Julie Weston. 2011. Continuous support for women during childbirth. *Cochrane Database of Systematic Reviews (online)* 2 (2) (Feb 16): CD003766.

Hofmeyr, G. Justus, Zarko Alfirevic, Anthony J. Kelly, Josephine Kavanagh, Jane Thomas, James P. Neilson, and Therese Downswell. 2009. Methods for cervical ripening and labour induction in late pregnancy: Generic protocol. *Cochrane Database of Systematic Reviews (online)* 3 (3) (July 8): CD002074.

Hofmeyr, G. Justus, A. Metin Gulmezoglu, and Cynthia Pileggi. 2010. Vaginal Misoprostol for cervical ripening and induction of labour. *Cochrane Database of Systematic Reviews (online)* 10 (10) (Oct 6): CD000941.

Hofmeyr, G. Justus, Jon F. Barrett, and Caroline A. Crowther. 2011. Planned caesarean section for women with a twin pregnancy. *Cochrane Database of Systematic Reviews (online)* 12 (12) (Dec 7): CD006553.

Hofmeyr, G. Justus, Mary Hannah, and Theresa Lawrie. 2010. Planned caesarean section for term breech delivery. *Cochrane Database of Systematic Reviews (online)* 1 (1) (Jan 20): CD000166.

Hofmeyr, G. Justus, and Regina Kulier. 2012. External cephalic version for breech presentation at term. *Cochrane Database of Systematic Reviews (online)* 10 (10) (Jan 29) :CD000083.

———. 2012. Operative versus conservative management for "fetal distress" in labour. *Cochrane Database of Systematic Reviews (online)* 6 (6) (June 13): CD001065.

Hofmeyr, G. Justus, and Theresa A. Lawrie. 2012. Amnioinfusion for potential or suspected umbilical cord compression in labour. *Cochrane Database of Systematic Reviews (online)* 1 (1) (Jan 18): CD000013.

Hutton, Eileen K., Angela H. Reitsma, and Karyn Kaufman. 2009. Outcomes associated with planned home and planned hospital births in low-risk women attended by midwives in Ontario, Canada, 2003–2006: A retrospective cohort study. *Birth (Berkeley, CA)* 36 (3) (Sep): 180–89.

Hyams, Andrew L., Jennifer A. Brandenburg, Stuart R. Lipsitz, David W. Shapiro, and Troyen A. Brennan. 1995. Practice guidelines and malpractice litigation: A two-way street. *Annals of Internal Medicine* 122 (6) (Mar 15): 450–55.

International Cesarean Awareness Network. 2012. VBAC hospitals in U.S. hospitals. Available at http://ican-online.org/vbac-ban-info (accessed January 26, 2013).

Irion, Olivier, and Michel Boulvain. 2009. Induction of labour for suspected fetal macrosomia. *Cochrane Database of Systematic Reviews (online)* 2 (2) (Oct 7): CD000938.

Jaffee, David. 2001. *Organizational theory: Tensions and change.* New York: Mc-Graw-Hill Higher Education.

Jain, Lucky, and Golde G. Dudell. 2006. Respiratory transition in infants delivered by cesarean section. *Seminars in Perinatology* 30 (5) (Oct): 296–304.

Janis, Irving L. 1971. Groupthink. *Psychology Today* 5 (6) (Nov): 43–46.

Jena, Anupam B., Seth Seabury, Darius Lakdawalla, and Amitabh Chandra. 2011. Malpractice risk according to physician specialty. *New England Journal of Medicine* 365 (7): 629–36.

Johnstone, F. D., R. J. Prescott, J. M. Steel, J. H. Mao, S. Chambers, and N. Muir. 1996. Clinical and ultrasound prediction of macrosomia in diabetic pregnancy. *BJOG: An International Journal of Obstetrics and Gynaecology* 103 (8) (Aug): 747–54.

Jordan, Brigitte. 1997. Authoritative knowledge and its construction. In *Childbirth and authoritative knowledge: Cross-cultural perspectives*, ed. Robbie E. Davis-Floyd and Carolyn F. Sargent, 55–79. Berkeley: University of California Press.

Jukelevics, Nicette. 2009. Putting mothers and babies at risk: Promoting the elusive "cesarean delivery on maternal request." *Birth (Berkeley, CA)* 36 (3) (Sep): 254–57.

Kachalia, Allen, Niteesh K. Choudhry, and David M. Studdert. 2005. Physician responses to the malpractice crisis: From defense to offense. *Journal of Law, Medicine, and Ethics: A Journal of the American Society of Law, Medicine, and Ethics* 33 (3) (Fall): 416–28.

Kalish, Robin B., Laurence B. McCullough, and Frank A. Chervenak. 2008. Patient choice cesarean delivery: Ethical issues. *Current Opinion in Obstetrics and Gynecology* 20 (2) (Apr): 116–19.

Kamal, Pallavi, Mary Dixon-Woods, Jennifer J. Kurinczuk, Christina Oppenheimer, Patricia Squire, and Jason Waugh. 2005. Factors influencing repeat caesarean section: Qualitative exploratory study of obstetricians' and midwives' accounts. *BJOG: An International Journal of Obstetrics and Gynaecology* 112 (8) (Aug): 1054–60.

Kennell, John, Marshall Klaus, Susan McGrath, Steven Robertson, and Clark Hinkley. 1991. Continuous emotional support during labor in a U.S. hospital: A randomized controlled trial. *JAMA: The Journal of the American Medical Association* 265 (17) (May 1): 2197–201.

Kesselheim, Aaron S., and David M. Studdert. 2006. Characteristics of physicians who frequently act as expert witnesses in neurologic birth injury litigation. *Obstetrics and Gynecology* 108 (2) (Aug): 273–79.

Khunpradit, Suthit, Pisake Lumbiganon, and Malinee Laopaiboon. 2011. Admission tests other than cardiotocography for fetal assessment during labour. *Cochrane Database of Systematic Reviews (online)* 6 (6) (Jun 15): CD008410.

Kingdon, C., J. Neilson, V. Singleton, G. Gyte, A. Hart, M. Gabbay, and T. Lavender. 2009. Choice and birth method: Mixed-method study of caesarean delivery for maternal request. *BJOG: An International Journal of Obstetrics and Gynaecology* 116 (7) (Jun): 886–95.

Klagholz, Jeffrey, and Albert L. Strunk. 2012. Overview of the 2012 ACOG survey on professional liability. Available from http://www.acog.org/About_ACOG/ACOG_Departments/Professional_Liability/2012_Survey_Results (accessed October 26, 2012).

———. 2009. Overview of the 2009 ACOG survey on professional liability. *ACOG Clinical Review.* Available from http://www.academia.edu/707493/Overview_of_the_2009_ACOG_survey_on_professional_liability (accessed October 26, 2012).

Klaus, Marshall H., John H. Kennell, Steven S. Robertson, and Roberto Sosa. 1986. Effects of social support during parturition on maternal and infant morbidity. *British Medical Journal (clinical research ed.)* 293 (6547) (Sep 6): 585–87.

Knight, Marian, Jennifer J. Kurinczuk, Patsy Spark, and Peter Brocklehurst, for the United Kingdom Obstetric Surveillance System Steering Committee. 2008. Cesarean delivery and peripartum hysterectomy. *Obstetrics and Gynecology* 111 (1) (Jan): 97–105.

Kohn, Linda T., Janet M. Corrigan, and Molla S. Donaldson, eds. 2000. *To err is human: Building a safer health system.* Washington, DC: National Academy Press.

Kotaska, Andrew. 2011. Commentary: Routine cesarean section for breech: The unmeasured cost. *Birth (Berkeley, CA)* 38 (2) (Jun): 162–64.

———. 2004. Inappropriate use of randomised trials to evaluate complex phenomena: Case study of vaginal breech delivery. *BMJ (clinical research ed.)* 329 (7473) (Oct 30): 1039–42.

Kotaska, Andrew J., Michael C. Klein, and Robert M. Liston. 2006. Epidural analgesia associated with low-dose oxytocin augmentation increases cesarean births: A critical look at the external validity of randomized trials. *American Journal of Obstetrics and Gynecology* 194 (3) (Mar): 809–14.

Kuehn, Bridget M. 2010. Expert panel calls for greater access to trial of labor after cesarean delivery. *JAMA: The Journal of the American Medical Association* 303 (17) (May 5): 1683–85.

Kuklina, Elena V., Susan F. Meikle, Denise J. Jamieson, Maura K. Whiteman, Wanda D. Barfield, Susan D. Hillis, and Samuel F. Posner. 2009. Severe obstetric morbidity in the United States, 1998–2005. *Obstetrics and Gynecology* 113 (2, pt. 1) (Feb): 293–99.

Lagan, Briege M., Marlene Sinclair, and W. George Kernohan. 2010. Internet use in pregnancy informs women's decision making: A web-based survey. *Birth (Berkeley, CA)* 37 (2) (Jun): 106–15.

Lagrew, David C., Jr., and Joseph A. Adashek. 1998. Lowering the cesarean section rate in a private hospital: Comparison of individual physicians' rates, risk factors, and outcomes. *American Journal of Obstetrics and Gynecology* 178 (6) (Jun): 1207–14.

Landon, Mark B. 2010. Predicting uterine rupture in women undergoing trial of labor after prior cesarean delivery. *Seminars in Perinatology* 34 (4) (Aug): 267–71.

———. 2008. Vaginal birth after cesarean delivery. *Clinics in Perinatology* 35 (3) (Sep): 491–504, ix–x.

Landon, Mark B., John C. Hauth, Kenneth J. Leveno, Catherine Y. Spong, Sharon Leindecker, Michael W. Varner, Atef H. Moawad, Steve N. Caritis, Margaret Harper, Ronald J. Wapner, Yoram Sorokin, Menachem Miodovnik, Marshall Carpenter, Alan M. Peaceman, Mary Jo O'Sullivan, Baha Sibai, Oded Langer, John M. Thorp, Susan M. Ramin, Brian M. Mercer, and Steve G. Gabbe, for the National Institute of Child Health and Human Development Maternal-Fetal Medicine Units Network. 2004. Maternal and perinatal outcomes associated with a trial of labor after prior cesarean delivery. *New England Journal of Medicine* 351 (25) (Dec 16): 2581–89.

Landon, Mark B., Catherine Y. Spong, Elizabeth Thom, John C. Hauth, Steven L. Gloom, Michael W. Varner, Atef H. Moawad, Steve N. Caritis, Margaret Harper, Ronald J. Wapner, Yoram Sorokin, Menachem Miodovnik, Marshall Carpenter, Alan M. Peaceman, Mary J. O'Sullivan, Baha M. Sibai, Oded Langer, John M. Thorp, Susan M. Ramin, Brian M. Mercer, and Steven G. Gabbe, for the National Institute of Child Health and Human Development Maternal–Fetal Medicine Units Network. 2006. Risk of uterine rupture with a trial of labor in women with multiple and single prior cesarean delivery. *Obstetrics and Gynecology* 108 (1) (Jul): 12–20.

Larsson, Christina, Karin Källen, and Ellika Andolf. 2009. Cesarean section and risk of pelvic organ prolapse: A nested case-control study. *American Journal of Obstetrics and Gynecology* 200 (3) (Mar): 243.e1–e4.

Leeman, Lawrence M., and Valerie J. King. 2011. Increasing patient access to VBAC: New NIH and ACOG recommendations. *American Family Physician* 83 (2) (Jan 15): 121–22, 127.

Leeman, Lawrence M., and Lauren A. Plante. 2006. Patient-choice vaginal delivery? *Annals of Family Medicine* 4 (3) (May/Jun): 265–68.

Levin, Myron. 2004. Injury claims face grueling fight: Victims increasingly view U.S. compensation program as adversarial and tightfisted. *Los Angeles Times,* November 29.

Liebhaber, Allison, and Joy M. Grossman. 2007. *Physicians moving to mid-sized, single-specialty practices.* Tracking Report 18. Washington, DC: Center for Studying Health System Change. Available from http://www.hschange.com/CONTENT/941/ (accessed January 31, 2013).

Lin, Herng-Ching, Tzong-Chyi Sheen, Chao-Hsiun Tang, and Senyeong Kao. 2004. Association between maternal age and the likelihood of a cesarean section: A population-based multivariate logistic regression analysis. *Acta Obstetricia et Gynecologica Scandinavica* 83 (12) (Dec): 1178–83.

Lin, Monique G. 2006. Umbilical cord prolapse. *Obstetrical and Gynecological Survey* 61 (4) (Apr): 269–77.

Little, Margaret Olivia, Anne Drapkin Lyerly, Lisa M. Mitchell, Elizabeth M. Armstrong, Lisa H. Harris, Rebecca Kukla, and Miriam Kuppermann. 2008. Mode of delivery: Toward responsible inclusion of patient preferences. *Obstetrics and Gynecology* 112 (4) (Oct): 913–18.

Little, Sarah E., Andrea G. Edlwo, Ann M. Thomas, and Nicole A. Smith. 2012. Estimated fetal weight by ultrasound: A modifiable risk factor for cesarean delivery? *American Journal of Obstetrics and Gynecology* 207 (4) (Oct): 309.e1–6.

Localio, A. Russell, Ann G. Lawthers, Joan M. Bengtson, Liesi E. Hebert, Susan L. Weaver, Troyen A. Brennan, and J. Richard Landis. 1993. Relationship between malpractice claims and cesarean delivery. *JAMA: The Journal of the American Medical Association* 269 (3) (Jan 20): 366–73.

Localio, A. Russell, Ann G. Lawthers, Troyen A. Brennan, Nan M. Laird, Liesi E. Hebert, Lynn M. Peterson, Joseph P. Newhouse, Paul C. Weiler, and Howard H. Hiatt. 1991. Relation between malpractice claims and adverse events due to negligence: Results of the Harvard Medical Practice Study III. *New England Journal of Medicine* 325 (4) (Jul 25): 245–51.

Luna, Zakiya. 2009. From rights to justice: Women of color changing the face of U.S. reproductive rights organizing. *Societies without Borders: Human Rights and the Social Sciences* 4: 343–65.

Lydon-Rochelle, Mona, Victoria L. Holt, Thomas R. Easterling, and Diane P.

Martin. 2001. Risk of uterine rupture during labor among women with a prior cesarean delivery. *New England Journal of Medicine* 345 (1) (Jul 5): 3–8.

Lyerly, Anne Drapkin, Lisa M. Mitchell, Elizabeth M. Armstrong, Lisa H. Harris, Rebecca Kukla, Miriam Kuppermann, and Margaret Olivia Little. 2007. Risks, values, and decision making surrounding pregnancy. *Obstetrics and Gynecology* 109 (4) (Apr): 979–84.

MacDorman, Marian F., Eugene Declercq, and T. J. Mathews. 2011. United States home births increase 20 percent from 2004 to 2008. *Birth (Berkeley, CA)* 38 (3) (Sep): 185–90.

MacDorman, Marian F., Eugene Declercq, Fay Menacker, and Michael H. Malloy. 2008. Neonatal mortality for primary cesarean and vaginal births to low-risk women: Application of an "intention-to-treat" model. *Birth (Berkeley, CA)* 35 (1) (Mar): 3–8.

MacDorman, Marian F., Fay Menacker, and Eugene Declercq. 2008. Cesarean birth in the United States: Epidemiology, trends, and outcomes. *Clinics in Perinatology* 35 (2) (Jun): 293–307.

Macones, George A., Alison G. Cahill, David M. Stamilio, Anthony Odibo, Jeffrey Peipert, and Erika J. Stevens. 2006. Can uterine rupture in patients attempting vaginal birth after cesarean delivery be predicted? *American Journal of Obstetrics and Gynecology* 195 (4) (Oct): 1148–52.

Macones, George A., Gary D. Hankins, Catherine Y. Spong, John Hauth, and Thomas Moore. 2008. The 2008 National Institute of Child Health and Human Development workshop report on electronic fetal monitoring: Update on definitions, interpretation, and research guidelines. *Obstetrics and Gynecology* 112 (3) (Sep): 661–66.

Macones, George A., Jeffrey Peipert, Deborah B. Nelson, Anthony Odibo, Erika J. Stevens, David M. Stamilio, Emmanuelle Pare, Michal Elovitz, Anthony Sciscione, Mary D. Sammel, and Sarah J. Ratcliffe. 2005. Maternal complications with vaginal birth after cesarean delivery: A multicenter study. *American Journal of Obstetrics and Gynecology* 193 (5) (Nov): 1656–62.

Makoha, F. W., H. M. Felimban, M. A. Fathuddien, F. Roomi, and T. Ghabra. 2004. Multiple cesarean section morbidity. *International Journal of Gynaecology and Obstetrics: The Official Organ of the International Federation of Gynaecology and Obstetrics* 87 (3) (Dec): 227–32.

Mangesi, L., G. J. Hofmeyr, and D. L. Woods. 2009. Assessing the preference of women for different methods of monitoring the fetal heart in labour. *South African Journal of Obstetrics and Gynaecology* 15 (2) (Aug): 58–59.

March, James G., and Herbert A. Simon. 1958. *Organizations*. New York: Wiley.

Marmor, Theodore R., and David M. Krol. 2002. Labor pain management in the United States: Understanding patterns and the issue of choice. *American Journal of Obstetrics and Gynecology* 186 (5, suppl.) (May): S173–80.

Martin, Joyce A., Brady E. Hamilton, Paul D. Sutton, Stephanie J. Ventura, Fay Menacker, and Sharon Kirmeyer. 2006. Births: Final data for 2004. *National Vital Statistics Reports* 55: 1–104.

Martin, Joyce A., Brady E. Hamilton, Stephanie J. Ventura, Michelle J. K. Osterman, Sharon Kirmeyer, T. J. Mathews, and Elizabeth Wilson. 2011. Births: Final data for 2009. *National Vital Statistics Reports* 60: 1–71.

Martin, Joyce A., Brady E. Hamilton, Stephanie J. Ventura, Michelle J. K. Osterman, Elizabeth Wilson, T. J. Mathews, and the Division of Vital Statistic. 2012. Births: Final data for 2010. *National Vital Statistics Report* 61: 1–71.

Martin, Karin. 2003. Giving birth like a girl. *Gender and Society* 17 (1): 54–72.

Matthews, Robert. 2000. Storks deliver babies (p=0.008). *Teaching Statistics* 22 (2): 36–38.

Mavroforou, Anna, Evgenios Koumantakis, and Emmanuel Michalodimitrakis. 2005. Physicians' liability in obstetric and gynecology practice. *Medicine and Law* 24 (1) (Mar): 1–9.

McCourt, Chris, Jane Weaver, Helen Statham, Sarah Beake, Jenny Gamble, and Debra K. Creedy. 2007. Elective cesarean section and decision making: A critical review of the literature. *Birth (Berkeley, CA)* 34 (1) (Mar): 65–79.

McGrath, Susan K., and John H. Kennell. 2008. A randomized controlled trial of continuous labor support for middle-class couples: Effect on cesarean delivery rates. *Birth (Berkeley, CA)* 35 (2) (Jun): 92–97.

McKinnie, Vikki, Steven E. Swift, Wei Wang, Patrick Woodman, Amy O'Boyle, Margie Kahn, Michael Valley, Deirdre Bland, and Joe Schaffer. 2005. The effect of pregnancy and mode of delivery on the prevalence of urinary and fecal incontinence. *American Journal of Obstetrics and Gynecology* 193 (2) (Aug): 512–18.

McMahon, Michael J., Edwin R. Luther, Watson A. Bowes Jr., and Andrew F. Olshan. 1996. Comparison of a trial of labor with an elective second cesarean section. *New England Journal of Medicine* 335 (10) (Sep 5): 689–95.

McNamara, Helen M., and Gary A. Dildy III. 1999. Continuous intrapartum pH, pO_2, pCO_2, and SpO_2 monitoring. *Obstetrics and Gynecology Clinics of North America* 26 (4) (Dec): 671–93.

Melamed, Nir, Yariv Yogev, Israel Meizner, Reuven Mashiach, and Avi Ben-Haroush. 2010. Sonographic prediction of fetal macrosomia. *Journal of Ultrasound in Medicine* 29 (2) (Feb): 225–30.

Mello, Michelle M. 2006. *Understanding medical malpractice insurance: A primer.* Robert Wood Johnson Foundation research synthesis report no. 8.

————. 2001. Of swords and shields: The role of clinical practice guidelines in medical malpractice litigation. *University of Pennsylvania Law Review* 149 (3) (Jan): 645–710.

Menacker, Fay, Marian F. MacDorman, and Eugene Declercq. 2010. Neonatal mortality risk for repeat cesarean compared to vaginal birth after cesarean (VBAC) deliveries in the United States, 1998–2002 birth cohorts. *Maternal and Child Health Journal* 14 (2) (Mar): 147–54.

Minkoff, Howard, and Dmitry Fridman. 2010. The immediately available physician standard. *Seminars in Perinatology* 34 (5) (Oct): 325–30.

Mitchell, Lisa Meryn. 2001. *Baby's first picture: Ultrasound and the politics of fetal subjects*. Toronto: University of Toronto Press.

Moffat, M. A., J. S. Bell, M. A. Porter, S. Lawton, V. Hundley, P. Danielian, and S. Bhattacharya. 2007. Decision making about mode of delivery among pregnant women who have previously had a caesarean section: A qualitative study. *BJOG: An International Journal of Obstetrics and Gynaecology* 114 (1) (Jan): 86–93.

Monari, Francesca, Simona Di Mario, Fabio Facchinetti, and Vittorio Basevi. 2008. Obstetricians' and midwives' attitudes toward cesarean section. *Birth (Berkeley, CA)* 35 (2) (June): 129–35.

Morris, Theresa, and Katherine McInerney. 2010. Media representations of pregnancy and childbirth: An analysis of reality television programs in the United States. *Birth (Berkeley, CA)* 37 (2) (Jun): 134–40.

Morrison, John C., Bonnie Flood Chez, Ian D. Davis, Rick W. Martin, William E. Roberts, James N. Martin Jr., and Randall C. Floyd. 1993. Intrapartum fetal heart rate assessment: Monitoring by auscultation or electronic means. *American Journal of Obstetrics and Gynecology* 168 (1, pt. 1) (Jan): 63–66.

Mozurkewich, E., J. Chilimigras, E. Koepke, K. Keeton, and V. J. King. 2009. Indications for induction of labour: A best-evidence review. *BJOG: An International Journal of Obstetrics and Gynaecology* 116 (5) (Apr): 626–36.

Murthy, Karna, William A. Grobman, Todd A. Lee, and Jane L. Holl. 2007. Association between rising professional liability insurance premiums and primary cesarean delivery rates. *Obstetrics and Gynecology* 110 (6) (Dec): 1264–69.

National Center for Injury Prevention and Control. 2011. WISQARS nonfatal injury reports. Available from http://webappa.cdc.gov/sasweb/ncipc/nfirates2001.html (accessed October 26, 2012).

Neilson, James P. 2012. Fetal electrocardiogram (ECG) for fetal monitoring during labour. *Cochrane Database of Systematic Reviews (online)* 4 (4) (April 18): CD000116.

Nelson, Karin B., James M. Dambrosia, Tricia Y. Ting, and Judith K. Grether. 1996.

Uncertain value of electronic fetal monitoring in predicting cerebral palsy. *New England Journal of Medicine* 334 (10) (Mar 7): 613–18.

Nilstun, Tore, Marwan Habiba, Göran Lingman, Rodolfo Saracci, Monica Da Frè, and Marina Cuttini for the EUROBS Study Group. 2008. Cesarean delivery on maternal request: Can the ethical problem be solved by the principlist approach? *Bio Med Central Medical Ethics* 9 (Jun 17): 11.

Nisenblat, Victoria, Shlomi Barak, Ofra Barnett Griness, Simon Degani, Gonen Ohel, and Ron Gonen. 2006. Maternal complications associated with multiple cesarean deliveries. *Obstetrics and Gynecology* 108 (1) (Jul): 21–26.

Oakley, Ann. 1986. *Captured womb: A history of the medical care of pregnant women.* Paperback ed. New York: Blackwell.

Oboro, Victor, Adeniyi Adewunmi, Anibaba Ande, Biodun Olagbuji, Michael Ezeanochie, and Ayodeji Oyeniran. 2010. Morbidity associated with failed vaginal birth after cesarean section. *Acta Obstetricia et Gynecologica Scandinavica* 89 (9) (Sep): 1229–32.

Ogbonmwan, S. E., V. Miller, D. E. Ogbonmwan, and A. A. Akinsola. 2010. Review of vaginal birth after primary caesarean section without prostaglandin induction and/or syntocinon augmentation in labour. *Journal of Maternal–Fetal and Neonatal Medicine: The Official Journal of the European Association of Perinatal Medicine, the Federation of Asia and Oceania Perinatal Societies, the International Society of Perinatal Obstetricians* 23 (4) (Apr): 281–85.

Osborne, Cara, Jeffrey L. Ecker, Kimberlee Gauvreau, and Ellice Lieberman. 2012. First-birth cesarean and risk of antepartum fetal death in a subsequent pregnancy. *Journal of Midwifery and Women's Health* 57 (1) (Jan/Feb): 12–17.

O'Shea, T. Michael, Mark A. Klebanoff, and Caroline Signore. 2010. Delivery after previous cesarean: Long-term outcomes in the child. *Seminars in Perinatology* 34 (4) (Aug): 281–92.

Ouzounian, Joseph G., David A. Miller, Christy J. Hiebert, Leah R. Battista, and Richard H. Lee. 2011. Vaginal birth after cesarean section: Risk of uterine rupture with labor induction. *American Journal of Perinatology* 28 (8) (Sep): 593–96.

Palmer, Donald. 1983. Broken ties: Interlocking directorates and intercorporate coordination. *Administrative Science Quarterly* 28 (1) (Mar): 40–55.

Parer, Julian T., and Tomoaki Ikeda. 2007. A framework for standardized management of intrapartum fetal heart rate patterns. *American Journal of Obstetrics and Gynecology* 197 (1) (Jul): 26.e1–e6.

Parry, Samuel, Christopher P. Severs, Harish M. Sehdev, George A. Macones, Laurel M. White, and Mark A. Morgan. 2000. Ultrasonograhic prediction of fetal macrosomia: Association with cesarean delivery. *Journal of Reproductive Medicine* 45 (1): 17–22.

Patel, Roshni R., Tim J. Peters, Deirdre J. Murphy, and the ALSPAC Study Team. 2005. Prenatal risk factors for caesarean section: Analyses of the ALSPAC cohort of 12,944 women in England. *International Journal of Epidemiology* 34 (2) (Apr): 353–67.

Paul, Pamela. 2009. The trouble with repeat cesareans. *Time*. February 19.

Pearlman, Mark D., and Paul A. Gluck. 2005. Medical liability and patient safety: Setting the proper course. *Obstetrics and Gynecology* 105 (5, pt. 1) (May): 941–43.

Perl, Lawrence M. 2010. The birth and death of VBACs in a rural community hospital. *Birth (Berkeley, CA)* 37 (3) (Sep): 257–58.

Perlow, Jordan H., Thomas Wigton, Jan Hart, Howard T. Strassner, Michael P. Nageotte, and Bradley M. Wolk. 1996. Birth trauma: A five-year review of incidence and associated perinatal factors. *Journal of Reproductive Medicine* 41 (10) (Oct): 754–60.

Petchesky, Rosalind Pollack. 1987. Fetal images: The power of visual culture in the politics of reproduction. *Feminist Studies* 13 (2) (Summer): 263–92.

Pettker, Christian M., and Charles J. Lockwood. 2008. New standards for FHR assessment: Something old and something new. *Contemporary OB/GYN* 53 (12): 10–12.

Pettker, Christian M., Stephen F. Thung, Errol R. Norwitz, Catalin S. Buhimschi, Cheryl A. Raab, Joshua A. Copel, Edward Kuczynski, Charles J. Lockwood, and Edmund F. Funai. 2009. Impact of a comprehensive patient safety strategy on obstetric adverse events. *American Journal of Obstetrics and Gynecology* 200 (5) (May): 492.e1–e8.

Pfeffer, Jeffrey, and Phillip Nowak. 1976. Joint ventures and interorganizational interdependence. *Administrative Science Quarterly* 21 (3) (Sep): 398–418.

Pfeffer, Jeffrey, and Gerald R. Salancik. 2003. *External control of organizations a resource dependence perspective*. Stanford business classics. Stanford, CA: Stanford Business Books.

Placek, Paul J., and Selma M. Taffel. 1988. Vaginal birth after cesarean (VBAC) in the 1980s. *American Journal of Public Health* 78 (5) (May): 512–15.

Podulka, Jennifer, Elizabeth Stranges, and Claudia Steiner. 2011. Hospitalizations related to childbirth, 2008. HCUP statistical brief no. 110 (Apr 2011). Agency for Healthcare Research and Quality. Rockville, MD. Available from http://www.hcup-us.ahrq.gov/reports/statbriefs/sb110.jsp (accessed October 26, 2012).

Press, Joshua Z., Michael C. Klein, Janusz Kaczorowski, Robert M. Liston, and Peter von Dadelszen. 2007. Does cesarean section reduce postpartum urinary incontinence? A systematic review. *Birth (Berkeley, CA)* 34 (3) (Sep): 228–37.

Quinn, Tristan. 2005. *Dead mums don't cry.* DVD, Bullfrog Films. Available from http://www.bullfrogfilms.com/catalog/dmdc.html (accessed October 26, 2012).

Ransom, Scott B., David M. Studdert, Mitchell P. Dombrowski, Michelle M. Mello, and Troyen A. Brennan. 2003. Reduced medicolegal risk by compliance with obstetric clinical pathways: A case-control study. *Obstetrics and Gynecology* 101 (4) (Apr): 751–55.

Reime, Birgit, Michael C. Klein, Ann Kelly, Nancy Duxbury, Lee Saxell, Robert Liston, Frédérique Josephine Petra Maria Prompers, Robert Stefan Willem Entjes, and Victor Wang. 2004. Do maternity care provider groups have different attitudes towards birth? *BJOG: An International Journal of Obstetrics and Gynaecology* 111 (12) (Dec): 1388–93.

Ritzer, George. 2004. *The McDonaldization of society.* Rev. ed. Thousand Oaks, CA: Pine Forge Press.

Roberts, Richard G., Mark Deutchman, Valerie J. King, George E. Fryer, and Thomas J. Miyoshi. 2007. Changing policies on vaginal birth after cesarean: Impact on access. *Birth (Berkeley, CA)* 34 (4) (Dec): 316–22.

Robinson, Barrett. 2008. A review of the proceedings from the 2008 NICHD workshop on the standardized nomenclature for cardiotocography. *Reviews in Obstetrics and Gynecology* 1 (2): 56–60.

Robinson, James C. 1999. *Corporate practice of medicine competition and innovation in health care.* California/Milbank series on health and the public. Berkeley: University of California Press.

Rock, Steven M. 1993. Variability and consistency of rates of primary and repeat cesarean sections among hospitals in two states. *Public Health Reports (Washington DC, 1974)* 108 (4) (Jul/Aug): 514–16.

———. 1988. Malpractice premiums and primary cesarean section rates in New York and Illinois. *Public Health Reports (Washington DC, 1974)* 103 (5) (Sep/Oct): 459–63.

Rollins, Mark, and Jennifer Lucero. 2012. Overview of anesthetic considerations for cesarean delivery. *British Medical Bulletin* 101: 105–25.

Rooks, Judith P. 2009. Oxytocin as a "high alert medication": A multilayered challenge to the status quo. *Birth (Berkeley, CA)* 36 (4) (Dec): 345–48.

Rortveit, Guri, Jeanette S. Brown, David H. Thom, Stephen K. Van Den Eeden, Jennifer M. Creasman, and Leslee L. Subak. 2007. Symptomatic pelvic organ prolapse: Prevalence and risk factors in a population-based, racially diverse cohort. *Obstetrics and Gynecology* 109 (6) (Jun): 1396–403.

Rosenthal, Sara M. 2006. Socioethical issues in hospital birth: Troubling tales from a Canadian sample. *Sociological Perspectives* 49 (3) (Fall): 369–90.

Roth, Rachel. 2000. *Making women pay: The hidden costs of fetal rights*. Ithaca: Cornell University Press.

Rouse, Dwight J., and John Owen. 1999. Prophylactic cesarean delivery for fetal macrosomia diagnosed by means of ultrasonography: A Faustian bargain? *American Journal of Obstetrics and Gynecology* 181 (2) (Aug): 332–38.

Rozen, Genia, Antony M. Ugoni, and Penny M. Sheehan. 2011. A new perspective on VBAC: A retrospective cohort study. *Women and Birth: Journal of the Australian College of Midwives* 24 (1) (Mar): 3–9.

Sacks, David A., and Wansu Chen. 2000. Estimating fetal weight in the management of macrosomia. *Obstetrical and Gynecological Survey* 55 (4) (Apr): 229–39.

Sakala, Carol, and Maureen P. Corry. 2008. *Evidence-based maternity care: What it is and what it can achieve*. New York: Milbank Memorial Fund.

Sakala, Carol, Suzanne F. Delbanco, and Harold D. Miller. 2013. The cost of having a baby in the United States. *Truven Health Analytics Marketscan Study*. Available from http://www.childbirthconnection.org/ (accessed February 1, 2013).

Sakala, Carol, Y. Tony Yang, and Maureen P. Corry. 2013. *Maternity care and liability: Pressing problems, substantive solutions*. New York: Childbirth Connection. Available from http://transform.childbirthconnection.org/reports/liability/ (accessed February 1, 2013).

Salam, Muhammad T., Helene G. Margolis, Rob McConnell, James A. McGregor, Edward L. Avol, and Frank D. Gilliland. 2006. Mode of delivery is associated with asthma and allergy occurrences in children. Annals of Epidemiology 16 (5) (May): 341–46.

Samuelsson, Eva C., F. T. Arne Victor, Gösta Tibblin, and Kurt F. Svardsudd. 1999. Signs of genital prolapse in a Swedish population of women 20 to 59 years of age and possible related factors. *American Journal of Obstetrics and Gynecology* 180 (2, pt. 1) (Feb): 299–305.

Sandelowski, Margarete. 1994. Separate, but less unequal: Fetal ultrasonography and the transformation of expectant mother/fatherhood. *Gender and Society* 8 (2) (Jun): 230–45.

Schneider, Mary Ellen. 2005. Insurers set criteria for VBAC coverage. *Ob.Gyn. News* 40 (3) (Feb 1): 1–2.

Schroeder, Elizabeth, Stavros Pedrou, Nishma Patel, Jennifer Hollowell, David Puddicombe, Maggie Redshaw, and Peter Brocklehurst. 2012. Cost effectiveness of alternative planned places of birth in woman at low risk of complications: Evidence from the Birthplace in England national prospective cohort study. *BMJ* 344 (e2292): 1–13.

Schutte, Joke M., Eric A. P. Steegers, Job G. Santema, Nico W. E. Schuitemaker, Jos van Roosmalen, and Maternal Mortality Committee of the Netherlands Society of Obstetrics. 2007. Maternal deaths after elective cesarean section for breech presentation in the Netherlands. *Acta Obstetricia et Gynecologica Scandinavica* 86 (2): 240–43.

Scifres, Christina M., Amanda Rohn, Anthony Odibo, David Stamilio, and George A. Macones. 2011. Predicting significant maternal morbidity in women attempting vaginal birth after cesarean section. *American Journal of Perinatology* 28 (3) (Mar): 181–86.

Scott, James R. 2010. Solving the vaginal birth after cesarean dilemma. *Obstetrics and Gynecology* 115 (6) (Jun): 1112–13.

Shaw-Battista, Jenna, Annette Fineberg, Barbara Boehler, Blanche Skubic, Deborah Wooley, and Zoe Titon. 2011. Obstetrician and midwife collaboration: Successful public health and private practice partnership. *Obstetrics and Gynecology* 118 (3) (Sept): 663–72.

Shea, Kevin G., Kevin J. Scanlan, Kurt J. Nilsson, Brent Wilson, and Charles Mehlman. 2008. Interstate variability of the statute of limitations for medical liability: A cause for concern? *Journal of Pediatric Orthopaedics* 28 (3) (Apr/May): 370–74.

Shi, Leiyu, and Douglas A. Singh. 2012. *Delivering health care in America: A systems approach.* 5th ed. Burlington, MA: Jones and Bartlett Learning.

Shihady, Ida R., Paula Broussard, Linda Burnes Bolton, Arlene Fink, Moshe Fridman, Rachel Fridman, Carolyn Aydin, Lisa M. Korst, and Kimberly D. Gregory. 2007. Vaginal birth after cesarean: Do California hospital policies follow national guidelines? *Journal of Reproductive Medicine* 52 (5) (May): 349–58.

Shortell, Stephen M. 2000. *Remaking health care in America: Building organized delivery systems.* 2nd ed. San Francisco: Jossey-Bass.

Siegal, Gil, Michelle M. Mello, and David M. Studdert. 2008. Adjudicating severe birth injury claims in Florida and Virginia: The experience of a landmark experiment in personal injury compensation. *American Journal of Law and Medicine* 34 (4): 493–537.

Silliman, Jael, Marlene Gerber Fried, Loretta Ross, and Elena Gutierrez. 2004. *Undivided rights: Women of color organize for reproductive justice.* Cambridge, MA: South End Press.

Silver, Robert M. 2010. Delivery after previous cesarean: Long-term maternal outcomes. *Seminars in Perinatology* 34 (4) (Aug): 258–66.

Simkin, Penny P., and MaryAnn O'Hara. 2002. Nonpharmacologic relief of pain during labor: Systematic reviews of five methods. *American Journal of Obstetrics and Gynecology* 186 (5, suppl.) (May): S131–59.

Simon, Herbert A. 1976. Administrative behavior: A study of decision-making processes in administrative organization. New York: Free Press.

Simonds, Wendy, Barbara Katz Rothman, and Bari Meltzer Norman. 2007. Laboring on: Birth in transition in the United States. Perspectives on gender. New York: Routledge.

Singata, Mandisa, Joan Tranmer, and Gillian M. L. Gyte. 2010. Restricting oral fluid and food intake during labour. Cochrane Database of Systematic Reviews (online) 1 (1) (Jan 20): CD003930.

Sipe, Theresa Ann, Judith T. Fullerton, and Kerri Durnell Schuiling. 2009. Nurse–midwives, certified nurse anesthetists, and nurse practitioners: Reflections on implications for uniform education and regulation. Journal of Professional Nursing 25 (3) (May/Jun): 178–85.

SisterSong Women of Color Reproductive Justice Collective. 2012. What is RJ? Available from http://www.sistersong.net/ (accessed February 27, 2012).

Sloan, Frank A., and Lindsey Chepke. 2008. Medical malpractice. Cambridge: MIT Press.

Sloan, Frank A., Stephen S. Entman, Bridget A. Reilly, Cheryl A. Glass, Gerald B. Hickson, and Harold H. Zhang. 1997. Tort liability and obstetricians' care levels. International Review of Law and Economics 17 (2): 245–60.

Smart, Derek R. 2012. Physician characteristics and distribution in the U.S., 2012. Chicago: American Medical Association.

Smith, Andrea. 2005. Beyond pro-choice versus pro-life: Women of color and reproductive justice. National Women's Studies Association Journal 17 (1) (Spring): 119–40.

Smith, Gordon C. S., Jill P. Pell, Alan D. Cameron, and Richard Dobbie. 2002. Risk of perinatal death associated with labor after previous cesarean delivery in uncomplicated term pregnancies. JAMA: The Journal of the American Medical Association 287 (20) (May 22–29): 2684–90.

Smith, James F., Cesar Hernandez, and Joseph R. Wax. 1997. Fetal laceration injury at cesarean delivery. Obstetrics and Gynecology 90 (3) (Sep): 344–46.

Smyth, Rebecca M. D., S. Kate Alldred, and Carolyn Markham. 2007. Amniotomy for shortening spontaneous labour. Cochrane Database of Systematic Reviews (online) 4 (4) (Oct 17): CD006167.

Sokol, Robert J., Sean C. Blackwell, and American College of Obstetricians and Gynecologists. Committee on Practice Bulletins—Gynecology. 2003. ACOG practice bulletin no. 40: Shoulder dystocia. International Journal of Gynaecology and Obstetrics: The Official Organ of the International Federation of Gynaecology and Obstetrics 80 (1) (Jan): 87–92.

Song, Felicia Wu, Jennifer Ellis West, Lisa Lundy, and Nicole Smith Dahmen.

2012. Women, pregnancy, and health information online: The making of informed patients and ideal mothers. *Gender and Society* 26 (5): 773–98.

Spencer, John. A. D., Nadia Badawi, Paul Burton, John Keogh, Patrick Pemberton, and Fiona Stanley. 1997. The intrapartum CTG prior to neonatal encephalopathy at term: A case-control study. *BJOG: An International Journal of Obstetrics and Gynaecology* 104 (1) (Jan): 25–28.

Spong, Catherine Y., Vincenzo Berghella, Katharine D. Wenstrom, Brian Mercer, and George R. Saade. 2012. Preventing the first cesarean delivery: Summary of a joint Eunice Kennedy Shriver National Institute of Child Health and Human Development, Society for Maternal-Fetal Medicine, and American College of Obstetricians and Gynecologists Workshop. *Obstetrics and Gynecology* 120 (5) (Nov): 1181–93.

Stapleton, Susan Rutledge, Cara Osborne, and Jessica Illuzzi. 2013. Outcomes of care in birth centers: Demonstration of a durable model. *Journal of Midwifery and Women's Health (online)* (Jan 30): 1–12.

Starr, Paul. 1982. *Social transformation of American medicine.* ACLS humanities e-book. New York: Basic Books.

State of Connecticut Insurance Department. 2009. Review of professional liability insurance rates. Available from http://www.ct.gov/cid/cwp/view.asp?Q=435460&A=3307 (accessed October 26, 2012).

Stevens, Rosemary. 1989. *In sickness and in wealth: American hospitals in the twentieth century.* New York: Basic Books.

Studdert, David M., Michelle M. Mello, and Troyen A. Brennan. 2004. Medical malpractice. *New England Journal of Medicine* 350 (3) (Jan 15): 283–92.

Sturdevant, Matthew. 2011. Obstetrician held liable. *Hartford Courant,* May 26.

Taffel, Selma M., Paul J. Placek, and Teri Liss. 1987. Trends in the United States cesarean section rate and reasons for the 1980–85 rise. *American Journal of Public Health* 77 (8) (Aug): 955–59.

Tang, Chao-Hsiun, Ming-Ping Wu, Jin-Tan Liu, Herng-Ching Lin, and Chun-Chyang Hsu. 2006. Delayed parenthood and the risk of cesarean delivery: Is paternal age an independent risk factor? *Birth (Berkeley, CA)* 33 (1) (Mar): 18–26.

Taylor, Janelle S. 2008. *The public life of the fetal sonogram.* New Brunswick: Rutgers University Press.

Timmermans, Stefan, and Marc Berg. 2003. *The gold standard: The challenge of evidence-based medicine and standardization in health care.* Philadelphia: Temple University Press.

Torres, Jennifer M., and Raymond G. De Vries. 2009. Birthing ethics: What mothers, families, childbirth educators, nurses, and physicians should know about ethics of childbirth. *Journal of Perinatal Education* 18 (1): 12–24

Turner, Michael J., Michael Brassil, and Harry Gordon. 1988. Active management of labor associated with a decrease in the cesarean section rate in nulliparas. *Obstetrics and Gynecology* 71 (2) (Feb): 150–54.

Tussing, A. Dale, and Martha A. Wojtowycz. 1997. Malpractice, defensive medicine, and obstetric behavior. *Medical Care* 35 (2) (Feb): 172–91.

———. 1994. Health maintenance organizations, independent practice associations, and cesarean section rates. *Health Services Research* 29 (1) (Apr): 75–93.

———. 1993. The effect of physician characteristics on clinical behavior: Cesarean section in New York State. *Social Science and Medicine* 37 (10) (Nov): 1251–60.

———. 1992. The cesarean decision in New York State, 1986: Economic and noneconomic aspects. *Medical Care* 30 (6) (Jun): 529–40.

United Nations. 2012. *The millennium development goals report, 2012.* New York: United Nations. Available from http://www.un.org/millenniumgoals/reports. shtml (accessed January 31, 2013).

U.S. Department of Health and Human Services. 2010. National practitioner data bank in U.S. Department of Health and Human Services (online). Available from http://www.npdb-hipdb.hrsa.gov/ (accessed October 26, 2012).

U.S. Department of Health and Human Services Health Resources and Services Administration. 2010. The Registered nurse population: Findings from the 2008 national sample survey of registered nurses. Available from *http://bhpr. hrsa.gov/healthworkforce/rnsurveys/rnsurveyfinal.pdf* (accessed August 31, 2012).

U.S. National Institutes of Health. 2012. Fetal ST segment and T wave analysis in labor (STAN). Available from http://clinicaltrials.gov/ct2/show/ NCT01131260 (accessed January 26, 2013).

———. 1980. Cesarean childbirth. *Consensus Development Conference Statements* 3 (6): 1–30.

Usta, Ihab M., Elie M. Hobeika, Antoine A. Musa, Gaby E. Gabriel, and Anwar H. Nassar. 2005. Placenta previa-accreta: Risk factors and complications. *American Journal of Obstetrics and Gynecology* 193 (3, pt. 2) (Sep): 1045–49.

Villar, José., Guillermo Carroli, Nelly Zavaleta, Allan Donner, Daniel Wojdyla, Anibal Faundes, Alejandro Velazco, Vicente Bataglia, Ana Langer, Alberto Narváez, Eliette Valladares, Archana Shah, Liana Campodónico, Mariana Romero, Sofia Reynoso, Karla Simônia de Pádua, Daniel Giordano, Marius Kublickas, and Arnaldo Acosta, for the World Health Organization 2005 Global Survey on Maternal and Perinatal Health Research Group. 2007. Maternal and neonatal individual risks and benefits associated with caesarean delivery: Multicentre prospective study. *BMJ (clinical research ed.)* 335 (7628) (Nov 17): 1025–35.

Wagner, Brian, Natalie Meirowitz, Jalpa Shah, Deepak Nanda, Lori Reggio, Phyllis Cohen, Karen Britt, Leah Kaufman, Rajni Walia, Corinne Bacote, Martin L. Lesser, Renee Pekmezaris, Adiel Fleischer, and Kenneth J. Abrams. 2011. Comprehensive perinatal safety initiative to reduce adverse obstetric events. *Journal for Healthcare Quality* 34 (1) (Jan/Feb): 6–15.

Walsh, Jennifer M., Nandini Kandamany, Niamh Ni Shuibhne, Helen Power, John F. Murphy, and Colm O'Herlihy. 2011. Neonatal brachial plexus injury: Comparison of incidence and antecedents between 2 decades. *American Journal of Obstetrics and Gynecology* 204 (4) (Apr): 324.e1–e6.

Weaver, Jane J., Helen Statham, and Martin Richards. 2007. Are there "unnecessary" cesarean sections? Perceptions of women and obstetricians about cesarean sections for nonclinical indications. *Birth (Berkeley, CA)* 34 (1) (Mar): 32–41.

Weber, Max, and Edward Shils. 1949. *Max Weber on the methodology of the social sciences.* Glencoe, IL: Free Press.

Weimar, C. H., A. C. Lim, M. L. Bots, H. W. Bruinse, and A. Kwee. 2010. Risk factors for uterine rupture during a vaginal birth after one previous caesarean section: A case-control study. *European Journal of Obstetrics, Gynecology, and Reproductive Biology* 151 (1) (Jul): 41–45.

Wells, C. Edward. 2010. Vaginal birth after cesarean delivery: Views from the private practitioner. *Seminars in Perinatology* 34 (5) (Oct): 345–50.

Whiteman, Maura K., Elena Kuklina, Susan D. Hillis, Denise J. Jamieson, Susan F. Meikle, Samuel F. Posner, and Polly A. Marchbanks. 2006. Incidence and determinants of peripartum hysterectomy. *Obstetrics and Gynecology* 108 (6) (Dec): 1486–92.

Williams, Helen O. 2008. The ethical debate of maternal choice and autonomy in cesarean delivery. *Clinics in Perinatology* 35 (2) (Jun): 455–62, viii.

Wilson, P. D., R. M. Herbison, and G. P. Herbison. 1996. Obstetric practice and the prevalence of urinary incontinence three months after delivery. *British Journal of Obstetrics and Gynaecology: An International Journal of Obstetrics and Gynaecology* 103 (2) (Feb): 154–61.

World Health Organization. 2012a. Trends in maternal mortality 1990 to 2010. World Health Organization database (online). Available from http://www. who.int/reproductivehealth/publications/monitoring/9789241503631/en/index.html (accessed September 12, 2012).

———. 2012b. Mortality rates, infant, per 1,000 live births. Available at http:// data.worldbank.org/indicator/SP.DYN.IMRT.IN (accessed October 18, 2012).

————. 1985. Appropriate technology for birth. *Lancet* 2 (8452) (Aug 24): 436–37.

Wright, Jason D., Neha Pawar, Julie S. R. Gonzalez, Sharyn N. Lewin, William M. Burke, Lynn L. Simpson, Abigail S. Charles, Mary E. D'Alton, and Thomas J. Herzog. 2011. Scientific evidence underlying the American college of obstetricians and gynecologists' practice bulletins. *Obstetrics and Gynecology* 118 (3) (Sep): 505–12.

Xu, Xiao, Kristine A. Siefert, Peter D. Jacobson, Jody R. Lori, and Scott B. Ransom. 2008. The impact of malpractice burden on Michigan obstetrician–gynecologists' career satisfaction. *Women's Health Issues: Official Publication of the Jacobs Institute of Women's Health* 18 (4) (Jul/Aug): 229–37.

Yang, Y. Tony, Michelle M. Mello, S. V. Subramanian, and David M. Studdert. 2009. Relationship between malpractice litigation pressure and rates of cesarean section and vaginal birth after cesarean section. *Medical Care* 47 (2) (Feb): 234–42.

Yang, Q., S. W. Wen, L. Oppenheimer, X. K. Chen, D. Black, J. Gao, and M. C. Walker. 2007. Association of caesarean delivery for first birth with placenta praevia and placental abruption in second pregnancy. *BJOG: An International Journal of Obstetrics and Gynaecology* 114 (5) (May): 609–13.

Yeh, John, Jean Wactawski-Wende, James A. Shelton, and Jennifer Reschke. 2006. Temporal trends in the rates of trial of labor in low-risk pregnancies and their impact on the rates and success of vaginal birth after cesarean delivery. *American Journal of Obstetrics and Gynecology* 194 (1) (Jan): 144.

Young, Diony. 2006. "Cesarean delivery on maternal request": Was the NIH conference based on a faulty premise? *Birth (Berkeley, CA)* 33 (3) (Sep): 171–74.

Young, Thomas K., and Barbara Woodmansee. 2002. Factors that are associated with cesarean delivery in a large private practice: The importance of prepregnancy body mass index and weight gain. *American Journal of Obstetrics and Gynecology* 187 (2) (Aug): 312–20.

Zhang, Jun, James Troendle, Uma M. Reddy, S. Katherine Laughon, D. Ware Branch, Ronald Burkman, Helain J. Landy, Judith U. Hibbard, Shoshana Haberman, Mildred M. Ramirez, Jennifer L. Bailit, Matthew K. Hoffman, Kimberly D. Gregory, Victor I I. Gonzalez-Quintero, Michelle Kominiarek, Lee A. Learman, Christos G. Hatjis, and Paul van Veldhuisen, for the Consortium on Safe Labor. 2010. Contemporary cesarean delivery practice in the United States. *American Journal of Obstetrics and Gynecology* 203 (4) (Oct): 326.e1–e10.

Zhani, Elizabeth Eaken. 2011. The Joint Commission expands performance measurement requirements. Press release. (November 30). Available at http://www.jointcommission.org/the_joint_commission_expands_performance_measurement_requirements/ (accessed February 1, 2013).

Zinberg, Stanley. 2001. Vaginal delivery after previous cesarean delivery: A continuing controversy. *Obstetrics and Gynecology* 44 (3) (September 2001): 561–70.

Zwart, J. J., J. M. Richters, F. Ory, J. I. de Vries, K. W. Bloemenkamp, and J. van Roosmalen. 2009. Uterine rupture in the Netherlands: A nationwide population-based cohort study. *BJOG: An International Journal of Obstetrics and Gynaecology* 116 (8) (Jul): 1069–80

Index

93–94; delivery before 39 weeks, 154; measurement of gestational age, 16

Gestational diabetes, 90

Glezerman, Marek, 63

Goldberg, Holly, 151

Goodrick, Elizabeth, 20–21

Grand rounds, 77

Groupthink, 76

Gun control, 128

Habiba, M., 150

Hannah, Mary E., 62

Health care, standardization of, 23–25, 187n128, 189n15

Health insurance: Affordable Care Act, 173; coverage of home births, 158; denial of coverage or higher premiums after c-section, 15; doulas not paid for by, 164, 181n3; global fee for birth by, 50; in vitro fertilization not covered by, 136

Health Maintenance Organizations (HMOs), 20

Heart-rate decelerations, fetal, 8; late, 9; variable, 9

Heart rate monitoring, fetal, 6, 182n20; two technologies for, 8; variability in, 9–10. See also Cardiotocography; Doppler unit; Electronic fetal monitoring

Hep- or saline-lock, 7

HMOs. See Health Maintenance Organizations

Home births, 157–58, 171

Hospitals: admission into, 6–7; control systems in, 28, 56–57, 153; goals of, 22–25; organizational imperatives for, 106–7; on perinatal Care Core

Measures, 173; solutions for, 163–64; teaching compared to nonteaching, 21; Yale, 58. See also Organizations; Patient safety movement

Hypoxia (lack of oxygen), 8

Hysterectomies, 15, 120, 121, 142

ICAN. See International Cesarean Awareness Network

Immediately available, 113, 116, 117, 122, 123, 129, 132

Incisions, 5–6, 118

Induction of labor, 7, 88–95, 161, 182n22; diabetes and, 90, 91; drugs for, 7, 88; due dates and, 89–90, 92–94; emergency c-sections after, 90–91, 94–95; liability and, 92–94; LTMII survey on, 7, 91, 93; for macrosomic babies, 89–90, 156; medical inductions, 89–92; rates of, 182n22; reasons for, 89; risks of, 89; scheduled before 39 weeks gestation, 154; social inductions, 89, 92; spontaneous labor compared to, 89; in VBACs, 125

Infant mortality rate, 170

Information on labor and birth, 144–49; LTMII survey on, 144–45

Informed consent, 7, 146, 149–51, 161, 197n12, 197n39

Informed consent forms: for c-sections, 2, 197n39; for labor and birth, 7, 150, 197n39; for VBACs, 138–39

Injuries, 10, 16; birth injury compensation, 167–70; brachial plexus injuries, 13, 85–86; fetal lacerations, 16, 102; shoulder dystocia, 13, 85–86

Institute of Medicine (IOM), 58

About the Author

Theresa Morris is Professor of Sociology at Trinity College in Hartford, Connecticut, where she teaches courses on Reproduction, Gender, and Research Methods.

Lightning Source UK Ltd.
Milton Keynes UK
UKHW011103280922
409568UK00002B/247